AF784101

Benefits and Risks of HORMONAL CONTRACEPTION

Benefits and Risks of

HORMONAL CONTRACEPTION

Has the Attitude Changed?

Edited by A. A. Haspels and R. Rolland

The Proceedings of an International Symposium,
Amsterdam, 19th March, 1982

MTP PRESS LIMITED
International Medical Publishers
LANCASTER · BOSTON · THE HAGUE

Published in the
United Kingdom and Europe by
MTP Press Limited, Falcon House
Lancaster, England

British Library Cataloguing in Publication Data

Benefits and risks of hormonal contraception.
1. Oral contraceptives–Congresses
I. Haspels, A. A. II. Rolland, R.
613.9′432 RE137.5

ISBN-13: 978-94-011-6677-5 e-ISBN-13: 978-94-011-6675-1

DOI: 10.1007/978-94-011-6675-1

Published in the USA by MTP Press
A division of Kluwer Boston Inc
190 Old Derby Street
Hingham, MA 02043, USA

Library of Congress Cataloging in Publication Data

Main entry under title:

Benefits and risks of hormonal contraception.

Papers presented at the International Symposium on Benefits and Risks of Hormonal Contraception, held in Amsterdam on March 19, 1982.
Includes index.
1. Oral contraceptives–Congresses. 2. Oral contraceptives–Side effects–Congresses. 3. Oral contraceptives–Physiological effect–Congresses.
I. Haspels, A. A. II. Rolland, R. III. International Symposium on Benefits and Risks of Hormonal Contraception (1982: Amsterdam, Netherlands)
[DNLM: 1. Contraceptives, Oral–Congresses.
2. Contraceptives, Oral–Adverse effects–Congresses.

QV 177 B464 1982]
RG137.5.B45 1982 615′.766 82-4615

Copyright © 1982 MTP Press Limited
Softcover reprint of the hardcover 1st edition 1982

All rights reserved. No part of this publication may be reproduced, stored in a retrieval system, or transmitted in any form or by any means, electronic, mechanical, photocopying, recording or otherwise, without prior permission from the publishers.

Phototypesetting by Swiftpages Limited, Liverpool

Contents

List of Active Participants

Professor Dr. M. Breckwoldt
Direktor der Abteilung für
Klinische Endokrinologie
Universitäts-Frauenklinik Freiburg
Freiburg
Fed. Rep. of Germany

Professor Dr. M.H. Briggs
Professor of Human Biology
Deakin University
Victoria
Australia

Professor Dr. I.A. Brosens
Gynecological and Endocrinological Dept.
University of Leuven
Leuven
Belgium

Dr. L. Carlborg
Associate Professor of
Obstetrics and Gynecology
Lanssjukhuset
Halmstad
Sweden

Professor Dr. E. Diczfalusy
Professor of Reproductive
Endocrinology
Reproductive Endocrinology
Research Unit
Karolinska Institute
Stockholm
Sweden

Dr. J.H. Evans
Senior Endocrinologist
Royal Women's Hospital
Carlton, Victoria
Australia

Dr. U.J. Gaspard
Dept. of Obstetrics and Gynecology
State University of Liège
Liège
Belgium

Professor Dr. J. Hammerstein
Leiter der Abteilung für
Gynäkologische Endokrinologie,
Sterilität und Familienplanung der
Frauenklinik im Klinikum Steglitz
der Freien Universität Berlin
Berlin
Fed. Rep. of Germany

Dr. H. Hannse
Vorstandsmitglied der Schering Aktiengesellschaft
Berlin/Bergkamen
Berlin
Fed. Rep. of Germany

Professor Dr. A.A. Haspels
Department of Obstetrics and Gynecology
University Hospital
Utrecht
The Netherlands

Professor Dr. G.A. Hauser
Chefarzt der Frauenklinik des Kantonsspitals
Lucerne
Switzerland

Professor Dr. K. Irsigler
Leiter der 3. Medizinischen Abteilung für Stoffwechselerkrankungen
Wien
Austria

Professor Dr. U. Larsson-Cohn
Department of Obstetrics and Gynecology
University Hospital
Linköping
Sweden

Dr. Th. Neufeld
Facharzt für Gynäkologie und Geburtshilfe
Wien
Austria

Professor Dr. R. Rolland
Department of Obstetrics and Gynecology
University Hospital Sint Radboud
Nijmegen
The Netherlands

Professor Dr. H.-D. Taubert
Leiter der Abteilung für Gynäkologische Endokrinologie
Zentrum für Frauenheilkunde und Geburtshilfe
Frankfurt/Main
Fed. Rep. of Germany

Professor Dr. G. Winckelmann
Leiter der Abteilung für Hämostaseologie
Deutsche Klinik für Diagnostik
Wiesbaden
Fed. Rep. of Germany

Dr. R.A. Wiseman
Medical Director
Schering Chemicals Ltd.
Burgess Hill
England

Professor Dr. R. Wyss
Chef de Service de la Policlinique de Gynecologie et d'Obstétrique
Hôpital Cantonal
Genève
Switzerland

Dr. G. Zador
Associate Professor of
Obstetrics and Gynecology at the
University of Uppsala, Sweden
Area Medical Director
Essex Chemie
Lucerne
Switzerland

Chairman's Introduction

A. A. Haspels

It is with pleasure that I welcome you, on behalf of Professor Rolland and myself, to Amsterdam for this International Symposium on 'Benefits and Risks of Hormonal Contraception'.

As a means of family planning the pill is about 25 years old – a timespan which has been characterized by an enormous increase in public interest and concern with family health and family-planning.

Undoubtedly we have learned a lot over the last 25 years. As you see in Figure 1, in the seventies in Holland relatively more fertile women used the pill than in any other country in the world.

In 1974 new combination pills were introduced containing less than 50 μg of ethinyl estradiol. In 1981 50% of Dutch pill-users took a sub-50 (Figure 2). The same is true for the Scandinavian countries.

In our own University Clinic 95% of pill-users take a sub-50 pill; only 5% use a 50 μg pill on medical indication. This decrease in estrogen dosage, which is usually accompanied by a decrease of progestational component as well, has resulted in a decrease of thromboembolic disease.

Factors that are still important to consider are diabetes mellitus, hypertension, adipositas and smoking.

Good selection of patients together with the prescribing where possible of sub-50 pills may result in the numbers of complications and side-effects being close to those encountered in the control group.

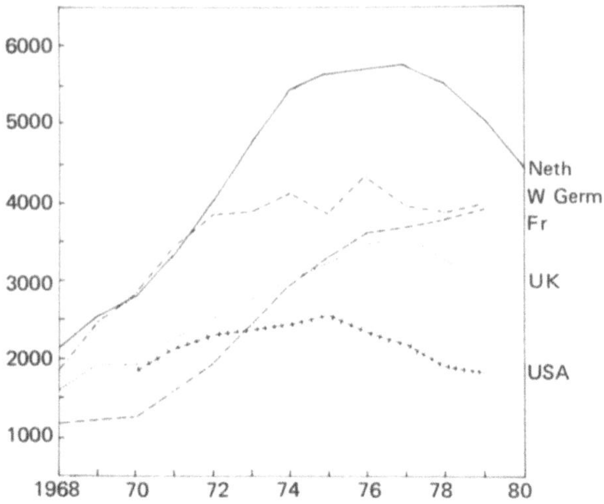

Figure 1 Number of pill-packs per 1000 fertile women aged 15–45

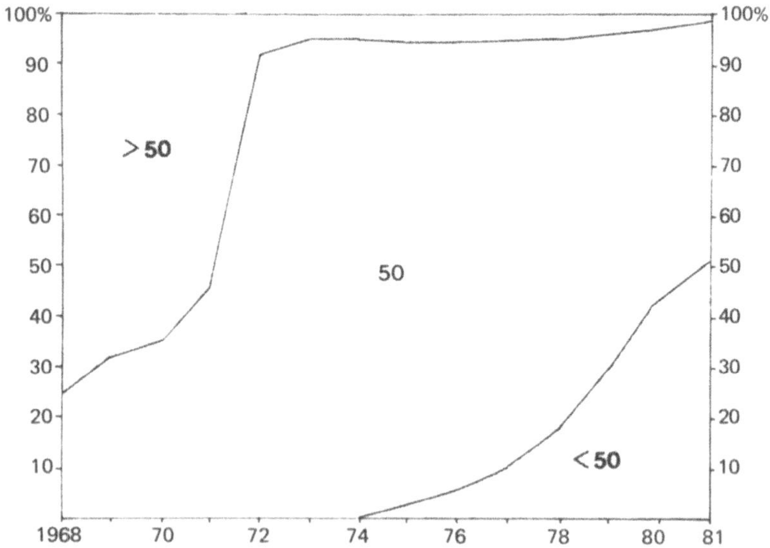

Figure 2 Combination pills – percentage with sub-50 μg estrogens

Most of the speakers today are actively engaged in contraceptive research and, from reading over their papers, it becomes clear that they have placed their work in the broader context of present day knowledge. It remains for me to mention how indebted we are to Schering, whose financial help made it possible to mount a conference of this quality!

Opening Remarks

H. Hannse

I have the pleasure of welcoming you on behalf of my colleagues from Schering AG to this international symposium. We appreciate it highly that you accepted our invitation to this meeting, sacrificing some of your precious time. I hope you will not be disappointed leaving this room tonight and not regret having come here.

Almost exactly 21 years ago our company, Schering AG, introduced the ovulation inhibitor Anovlar® in Australia. Anovlar represented the first hormone preparation to be developed in Europe especially for contraception. In the following 21 years a number of other hormonal contraceptives have been developed, ten of them alone by Schering AG. What kind of progress has this development produced and where are we today? The intention of this symposium is to give us a general picture of the accumulated experiences of more than two decades of research and development. I wish to thank in advance the moderators and speakers who are prepared to make a contribution to this symposium from the point of view of their special area. I am especially grateful that Professor Haspels and Professor Rolland have been willing to act as chairmen of this meeting. The 'Father of the Pill' is correctly deemed to be the American reproduction physiologist, Dr Gregory Pincus, who, together with the gynecologists Rock and Garcia, tested the principle of hormonal inhibition of ovulation in the years

1951–1958 and demonstrated its practicality with nearly 100% reliability in preventing conception.

The scientists of our company based their work on this experience when they developed Anovlar, using an highly effective progestogen synthesized in Berlin. If Schering AG was able to play the role of a pioneer in the realization of what was at the time a new biological principle for contraception, it was because Schering's researchers had already created important preconditions for doing so in the 1920s and 1930s. I include amongst these preconditions the investigation of the cybernetic mechanism of control in the endocrine system that makes it possible to prevent ovulation with progestogen–estrogen combinations. Members of our research departments like Hohlweg and Junkmann made a decisive contribution to the elucidation of this feedback mechanism.

After their isolation and purification, the structure of the female sexual hormones was explored and demonstrated by synthesis in cooperation with Schering AG by Professor Butenandt of Göttingen. The isolation of estrone succeeded in 1929 and that of progesterone in 1934. Butenandt was awarded the Nobel prize for these achievements in 1939. This advance made possible the large scale semisynthetic production of female hormones and their broad therapeutic use in the form of preparations like Progynon[R] and Proluton[R]. Concentrates and extracts made of biological material used until then could be replaced by exactly dosed preparations with constant efficacy.

In 1938, in our central laboratory at that time, Inhoffen and Hohlweg synthesized ethinyl estradiol that turned out to be a highly potent and, above all, orally effective estrogen and is still today the most important estrogen component of oral contraceptives worldwide. In the same year ethinyl testosterone, also called ethisterone, was synthesized. It is the parent substance of many ethinyl compounds of the 19-nor series which include the most important progestogen components of oral contraceptives used today. Norethisterone was the first to be synthesized by

Djerassi in 1951. Schering in Berlin took the step of creating norethisterone acetate, the progestogenic effect of which is clearly stronger than that of the basic substance. A decisive advance was the total synthesis of norgestrel by Hershel-Smith in 1961. Norgestrel is an enanthiomeric mixture of two components. With the help of microbiological methods and stereoselective chemical synthesis Schering succeeded in producing the pure levonorgestrel, the biologically effective component of this mixture which constitutes norgestrel. Today in hormonal contraception levonorgestrel is the most widely used oral progestogen.

Further contributions made by our company, Schering AG, to the development of fertility control were the so-called calendar packs which made the control of the daily intake of the pill much easier for women. The first pack with 21 coated tablets and the imprinted names of the individual days of the week was introduced in 1963 for application according to the plan '3 weeks on, one week off'. In 1964 there followed a pack with 28 coated tablets in the case of which the medication-free interval was bridged with seven placebos in order to avoid mistakes when starting a new pack after the break. In 1973 it was possible to introduce Microgynon[R] 30 as the first preparation with only 30 μg of EE per coated tablet, that is still today the lowest dose of the estrogen component in birth control pills. In our view the present ultimate in the optimization of hormonal contraceptives is represented by Triquilar[R], in which it was possible to reduce the total amount of sexual steroids required per cycle to a minimum, namely only 2.6 mg, while maintaining a reliable contraceptive effect! If you keep in mind that it started with 200 mg per cycle in the case of the Pincus preparation, that clearly shows what progress has been achieved in the last two decades.

After my opening remarks, let us learn how the balance of benefits and risks of hormonal contraception more than two decades after the introduction in the daily practice of medicine is judged by leading international experts. I open this symposium officially and pass the word to the moderator of the first session, Professor Breckwoldt!

Company Note
Triquilar[R] the triphasic pill developed by Schering is clinically proven in more than 20 000 documented cycles and in far more than 16 million user cycles in the short time since its availability. Other trade names are Trigynon[R], Logynon[R], Trionetta[R], Triagynon[R] and Trikvilar[R].

Section I

The Present Situation in General

Moderator: M. Breckwoldt

Chapter 1

What does it take to develop a new contraceptive?

E. Diczfalusy

Do we really need improved and new fertility regulating agents? This problem is debated mainly in the Western world, sometimes perhaps at a pleasant distance from reality. However, in developing countries the views are different and Vice Prime Minister Chen Mu-hua of the People's Republic of China[1] and Prime Minister Indira Gandhi[2], two ladies representing more than 40% of the population of the world, repeatedly urged intensified international efforts (especially through the services of the World Health Organization) to develop a large variety of safe and inexpensive fertility regulating agents.

Why do we need such a large variety of methods? Because – due to cultural, socio-economic and religious differences – certain methods are unacceptable to certain populations. Furthermore, different methods are needed for different age groups. Differences in the development of the health services represent another important reason. Moreover, the frequency of side-effects varies in different populations. Unexpected effects might be observed following long-term use of any method, and – because of the polymorphism of human populations – rare adverse effects may occur in a few specially sensitive individuals, using almost any method.

If there is such a great need for new methods, why don't we develop a large variety of them at once? Indeed, when the first oral contraceptive, Enovid[R], was developed, it took only some five years from the synthesis of a new chemical entity[3] to its marketing[4]. However, Edmund Burke said almost 200 years ago that 'you can never plan the future by the past'[5], and today the development of a new fertility regulating agent will take a minimum of 15–20 years and will cost some 50 million dollars[6-10].

Why does it take such a long time and so much money for a new chemical entity to reach the consumer in the form of a new fertility regulating drug? As Horatio said in his Art of Poetry, '*difficile est proprie communia dicere*'; the simple things are usually the most difficult to explain. Nevertheless, I will try, because it is important to understand what the prospects are for the next 15–20 years. So, what does it take to develop a new contraceptive, for instance a pill for men?

The most essential prerequisite is *basic research*, which requires strong support in order to generate new ideas and, indeed, one of our present problems is that support to the study of human reproduction considerably decreased during the past decade[11].

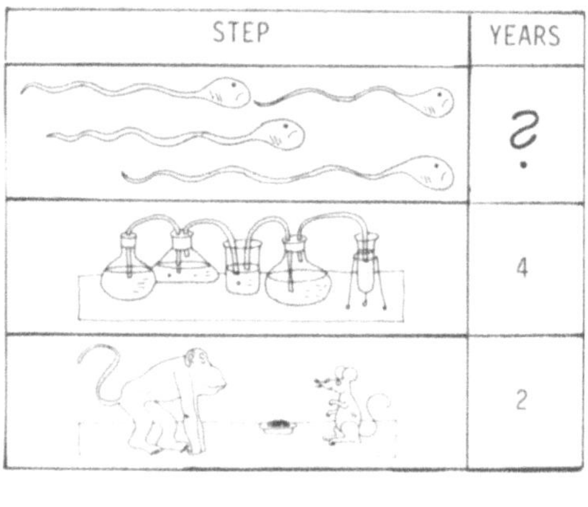

Figure 1 A hypothetical substance has been discovered, which selectively inhibits sperm motility. Several hundreds of analogues are synthesized and screened for efficacy. (After Diczfalusy (1978). Beyond the pill. *World Health*, August–September, reproduced by permission of the World Health Organization)

Let us assume now that – thanks to basic research – a new agent was discovered which selectively inhibits sperm motility (Figure 1). What is required to translate this finding into a widely available 'pill for men'? The first question that has to be answered is whether this is the best possible compound, or are there much better ones? To answer this, several hundred or perhaps a thousand related compounds (analogues) are synthesized and screened in suitable animal models for *efficacy*. Many serious problems are hidden beyond this simple statement; is the animal model really relevant? Does it permit valid extrapolation to the human? Is it feasible to use a given species in sufficient numbers, and will the time and cost be reasonable? A frequent compromise is to screen the compounds in a relatively inexpensive rodent, for instance in the rat, and then re-assess the efficacy of the most promising ones in another species, preferably a subhuman primate. Hence the work involved at this stage is considerable, and it may easily take 4–6 years before a favored compound can be selected for further development. Furthermore, although at this stage we are mainly concerned with *efficacy*, we must also conduct literature studies on the *safety* of previously described chemically related compounds, since reports on possible toxic manifestations by certain groups of compounds may influence the selection process.

When a compound has been selected, what next? First of all, it must be produced on a larger scale, in a pilot plant, because large quantities will be needed for the animal toxicological studies, which must be carried out before the drug can be given to human volunteers (Figure 2). Again, the scaling up of a synthetic procedure may be quite complicated and time-consuming.

The requirements for animal toxicological assessment will vary, not only with the type and proposed use of the compound, but also from country to country[10,12–14]. However, for a male contraceptive it will probably involve, at this stage, acute toxicity studies in at least two rodent and one non-rodent species

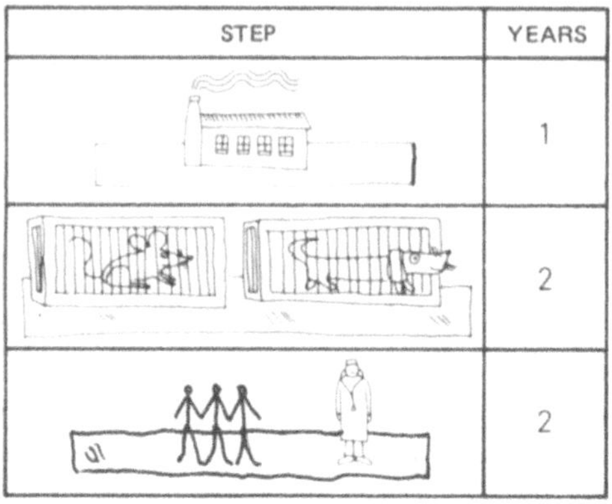

Figure 2 The most promising compound is synthesized on a larger scale and subjected to toxicological assessment in animals before clinical testing in a Phase I study. (Modified from Diczfalusy (1978). Beyond the pill. *World Health*, August–September, reproduced by permission of the World Health Organization)

and by two routes of administration; the one which is proposed for use in man, and another route, which must produce definite absorption. Since, furthermore, fertility regulating agents will be administered on several occasions, repeated dose studies must also be conducted – say, for 6 months – usually in one rodent and one non-rodent species, and at least at three dose levels (a) at the expected human dose, (b) at the maximum tolerated dose, and (c) at an even higher dose, which is so high that it must produce a toxic response. We have to know what types of toxic manifestations might arise if the drug is overdosed[22].

It goes without saying that the interpretation of the last group of findings is not an easy one and that the design of protocols for all toxicological studies is of crucial importance. For instance, in case the elimination of the drug from the organism of the animal is relatively slow, a too frequent administration of it at arbitrarily chosen intervals may lead to a gradual accumulation of the compound and its metabolites and may produce adverse effects of such a type which will perhaps never occur in man.

Hence, the importance of conducting simultaneous pharmacokinetic investigations on a satellite group of animals already at this early stage of development must be particularly underlined. Furthermore, the animal model selected for toxicological assessment may be inappropriate, and there is a danger that the results obtained may not be properly interpreted, unless sufficient pharmacodynamic information is available on similar drugs in the species in question. Indeed, the credit should go to Professor Friedmund Neumann and his co-workers at Schering AG, Berlin, who demonstrated that the beagle dog is an unsuitable model for the assessment of the safety of progestational agents, because, in contradistinction to what happens in other species (e.g. human, monkey, rat), the administration of progestogens (including the natural hormone, progesterone) induces hypersecretion of growth hormone, acromegaly and mammary nodules[15–17], which – following the administration of certain compounds, at least – may sometimes become malignant[18]. Indeed, the importance of growth hormone secretion for the induction of mammary growth in the canine species is further illustrated by the fact that high doses of a potent progestogen, cyproterone acetate (40 mg/kg daily p.o. for 8 weeks), did not cause any significant stimulation of mammary growth in hypophysectomized female beagle dogs (Neumann *et al.*, personal communication). It was on the basis of these mammary nodules that the Food and Drug Administration of the United States some 10 years ago banned a number of progestational steroids. What their view is today is not yet known; their previous view is certainly not shared by the Toxicology Review Panel of the World Health Organization[19]. At any rate, the lack of adequate pharmacokinetic and pharmacodynamic information on a compound in the toxicological model selected for the assessment of its safety may sometimes kill a valuable product.

If the animal toxicological evaluation goes very well, then the first clinical assessment may be started in the form of a Phase I study (Figure 2). In essence, the Phase I study is a human tolerance study; we administer a small dose once, or perhaps twice, to a very limited number of volunteers (say 3–5) in a hospital setting and look very carefully for unexpected effects. Nowadays, at this stage, a variety of laboratory analyses are also carried out in order to get some early information as to the likely behavior of the drug in human pharmacokinetic and pharmacodynamic studies[23].

However, a Phase I study cannot be carried out unless the protocols are approved by a number of Regulatory Agencies. For instance, as indicated in Figure 3, in the Special Programme of the World Health Organization the protocols must be approved by the Task Force Steering Committee, the Toxicology Review Panel, the Review Group and the Secretariat Committee for Research involving Human Subjects. However, the last mentioned Committee will not consider any protocols unless they have been approved previously by the National Drug

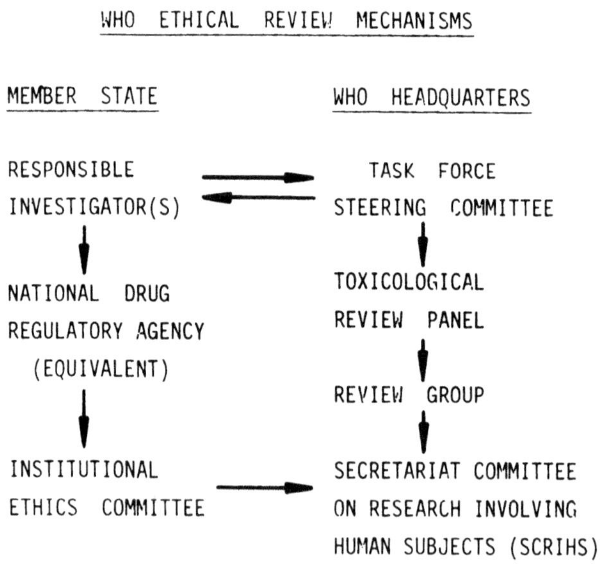

Figure 3 Technical and ethical review mechanisms in the Special Programme of the World Health Organization

Regulatory Agency and by a local Ethics Committee. The same procedure of approval will then be repeated prior to the initiation of Phase II and Phase III studies (see below).

If the Phase I study goes well, a Phase II investigation will be conducted on, say, 50–100 subjects (Figure 4). The purpose of the exercise is to establish the optimal dosage. However, before the Phase II study can be started, a great deal more animal toxicological assessment is required. Again, the regulations for this will vary from compound to compound and from country to country, but the likelihood is that for a new fertility regulating agent the authorities will request a 1–2 year toxicological assessment in three species, for instance rat, dog and monkey. Somewhat later, but before Phase III, it will also be necessary to conduct a number of special studies in one or two species on the effect of the drug on subsequent fertility, on perinatal and postnatal effects, and we must also carefully assess its teratogenic, mutagenic and carcinogenic potential[23].

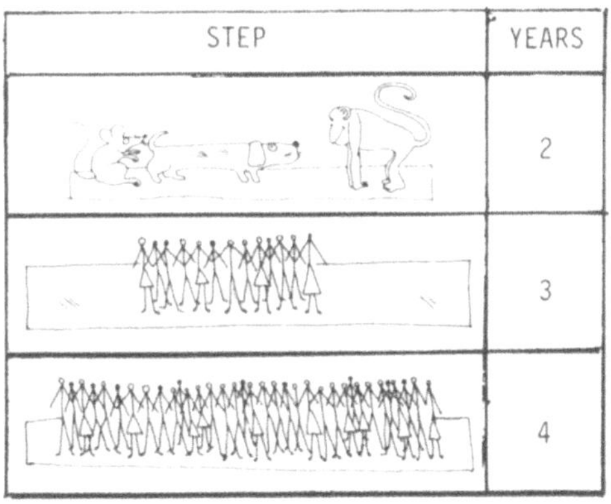

Figure 4 After two years toxicological study in several animal species, the new compound is tested in Phase II and Phase III studies. (Modified from Diczfalusy (1978). Beyond the pill. *World Health,* August–September, reproduced by permission of the World Health Organization)

Once the conditions discussed above are met, we can proceed to the Phase III study. This will be conducted in, say, up to 1000 subjects under field conditions and not in a hospital setting. Our main concern will be to establish the overall efficacy in real life and to look for rare adverse reactions.

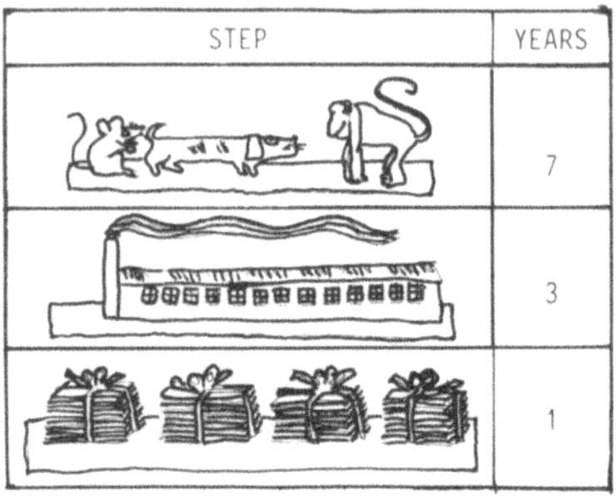

Figure 5 Simultaneously with the Phase III study, lifetime toxicological investigations are initiated. The new drug is manufactured on a large scale and the documentation is submitted for registration. (After Diczfalusy (1978). Beyond the pill. *World Health,* August–September, reproduced by permission of the World Health Organization)

However, before starting the Phase III study, in most Western countries one must initiate lifetime toxicological studies in two species, for instance 7 years in dogs and 10 years in monkeys (Figure 5). We do not have to complete these toxicological studies before embarking on the Phase III investigation, but it must be documented that they are ongoing and one has to submit periodical progress reports to the Regulatory Authorities. We must also conduct a large number of clinical studies, for instance on the bioavailability, mechanism of action and metabolic effects of the drug. Also, the synthetic method must again be scaled up to enable fabrication on a large scale. A number of formulation studies must also be conducted, together with prolonged tests of stability, for instance at elevated temperature and high humidity. Moreover, one must develop detailed specifications, suitable methods for quality control and compile a tremendous amount of documentation to be submitted for registration to the Drug Regulatory Authorities together with the results of the Phase III studies. By the time this is done, some 20 years have elapsed and several of the research workers who have initiated the project might have reached retirement age.

Of course, several of the steps indicated above can and should be carried out simultaneously, according to a critical path map shown in Figure 6, which is a somewhat simplified version[8] of the original example published by Djerassi[6]. In this hypothetical example, Djerassi calculated that the stage of registration would have been reached in 17 years. He was much criticized for this 'undue pessimism' by the optimists of that time. In retrospect it is easy to see now who was right. However, due to the human condition, professional optimists are the sacred cows of modern

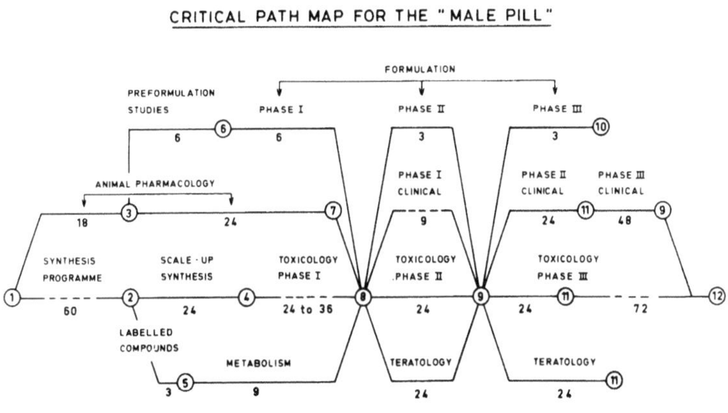

Figure 6 A simplified representation of a 'critical path map' (Diczfalusy[8]) published originally by Djerassi[6] to indicate the various steps (encircled figures) and time required for the development of a 'male pill'. The small figures below the various steps indicate the number of months required for the completion of that particular task

society and it is sacrilegious to remind them that they were wrong, although – in fact – undue optimism might interfere with progress in a field just as much as undue pessimism.

It should be emphasized that many drugs which are not contraceptive may be registered in a considerably shorter time, partly because much less animal toxicology is required; the differences are indicated in Table 1, taken from a paper by di Raddo & Wardell[10].

Table 1 Animal toxicological requirements for contraceptives and other drugs in the United States. (According to di Raddo & Wardell[10])

Toxicology	*Contraceptives*	*Other drugs*
Pre-phase I	Rat, dog, monkey 90 days	Two species 2–4 weeks
Pre-phase II	Rat, dog, monkey 1 year	Two species 90 days
Pre-phase III	Rat, dog, monkey 2 years + Lifetime studies initiated in dogs (7 years) and monkeys (10 years)	
NDA	Progress reports on the lifetime studies	Rat: 2 years Mouse: 18 months Dog: 1 year

Why is so much animal toxicology needed for new contraceptives? Because agents of this type will be administered to millions of healthy individuals during prolonged periods of time and with a minimum of medical supervision. From this it also follows that registration and marketing is not the end of the road; it is really the beginning, a new departure. From now on the epidemiologists will take over, and during many, many years to come we will carefully follow the major areas of continuous concern, such as neoplasia and various metabolic changes. We will look for endocrine effects, thromboembolic complications and changes in blood pressure after long-term exposure, and eventually will also assess possible second generation effects. Hence contraceptive drug development means to 'perform an act whereof what's past is prologue, what to come in yours and mine discharge'[20].

Finally, I would like to point out that during the period 1963–1976 almost 1000 new chemical entities reached the stage of clinical testing in the USA. Only 20 of these were fertility regulating agents. Furthermore, by 1976, the average cost of development for new fertility regulating agents exceeded 50 million dollars and the average patent life calculated from the time of NDA approval was reduced from 13.6 to 9.5 years[10].

Some 2300 years ago, Protagoras said that 'many things stand in the way of knowledge, the obscurity of the subject and the brevity of human life'. With apologies to Protagoras, as a late epigone, I will slightly modify the famous quotation by saying that many things stand in the way of contraceptive development: the complexity of the subject, the enormous cost and the brevity of patent life.

References

1. Chen Mu-Hua (1970). Realization of the four modernizations hinges on planned control of population growth. *The People's Daily*, *Beijing*, August 11th
2. Indira Gandhi (1981). Address to the World Health Assembly, May. A34/V4/ p. 19–22
3. Colton, F. B. (1955). 13-methyl-17-ethynyl-17-hydroxy-1,2,3,4,6,7,8, 9,11,12,13,14,16,17-tetradecahydro-15H-cyclo-penta(α)phenanthren-3-one and its preparation. U.S. Patent No. 2,725,389
4. Drill, V. A. (1966). *Oral Contraceptives*. (New York: The Blakiston Division, McGraw-Hill)
5. Burke, E. (1796). Letter to a Member of the National Assembly
6. Djerassi, C. (1970). Birth control after 1984. *Science*, **169**, 941
7. Djerassi, C. (1979). In *The Politics of Contraception*. p. 171. (Stanford, Calif.: Stanford Alumni Association)
8. Diczfalusy, E. (1979). Future methods of fertility regulation. *Int. J. Gynaecol. Obstet.*, **16**, 571
9. Diczfalusy, E. (1982). Gregory Pincus and steroidal contraception revisited. *Acta Obstet. Gynecol. Scand. Suppl.*, **105**, 7
10. di Raddo, I. and Wardell, W. M. (1981). Research activity on systemic contraceptive drugs by the US Pharmaceutical Industry. *Contraception*, **23**, 345

11. Greep, R. O., Koblinsky, M. A. and Jaffe, F. S. (1976). *Reproduction and Human Welfare: a Challenge to Research.* (Ford Foundation)
12. Overbeek, G. A., Hornstra, H. W., van Julsingha, E. B., Mumford, J. P. and Zayed, I. (1974). Special requirements for toxicity testing of oral compounds administered continuously or cyclically. In Briggs, M. H. and Diczfalusy, E. (eds.) Pharmacological Models in Contraceptive Development. *Acta Endocr. (Kbh.) Suppl.*, **185**, 387
13. Berliner, V. R. (1974). US Food and Drug Administration requirements for toxicity testing of contraceptive products. In Briggs, M. H. and Diczfalusy, E. (eds.) Pharmacological Models in Contraceptive Development. *Acta Endocr. (Kbh.) Suppl.* **185**, 240
14. Lerner, L. J. Special requirements for testing post-coital contraceptives. In Briggs, M. H. and Diczfalusy, E. (eds.) Pharmacological Models in Contraceptive Development. *Acta Endocr. (Kbh.) Suppl.* **185**, 355
15. El Etreby, M. F., Gräf, K.-J., Beier, S., Elger, W., Günzel, P. and Neumann, F. (1979). Suitability of the beagle dog as a test model for the tumorigenic potential of contraceptive steroids. A short review. *Contraception*, **20**, 237
16. El Etreby, M. F., Gräf, K.-J., Günzel, P. and Neumann, F. (1979). Evaluation of effects of sexual steroids on the hypothalamic-pituitary system of animals and man. *Arch. Toxicol.*, *Suppl.*, **2**, 11. (Berlin: Springer Verlag)
17. El Etreby, M. F. and Neumann, F. (1980). Influence of sex steroids and steroid antagonists on hormone dependent tumours in experimental animals. In Jacobelli, S. *et al.* (eds.) *Hormones and Cancer.* pp. 321–336. (New York: Raven Press)
18. Berliner, V. (1974). In Briggs, M. H. and Diczfalusy, E. (eds.) Pharmacological Models in Contraceptive Development. *Acta Endocr. (Kbh.) Suppl.*, **185**, 261
19. World Health Organization (1982). Facts about injectable contraceptives. *Bull. WHO*, **60**, 199
20. Shakespeare, W. *The Tempest.* II, I
21. Diczfalusy, E. (1978). Beyond the pill. *World Health*, August–September. pp. 22–25
22. Noel, P. R. B. (1974). Traditional animal screening tests. In Briggs, M. H. and Diczfalusy, E. (eds.) Pharmacological Models in Contraceptive Development. *Acta Endocr. (Kbh). Suppl.* **185**, 17
23. Briggs, M. H. and Diczfalusy, E. (eds.) (1974). Pharmacological Models in Contraceptive Development. *Acta Endocr. (Kbh). Suppl.* **185**, 1

Chapter 2

Influence of mass media on the attitude towards oral contraceptives

G. A. Hauser

During the first 10 years in which ovulation inhibitors were used the great variation in the incidence of side-effects of these preparations attracted our attention (Figure 1). However, an analysis of these side-effects, by preparations used, (Figure 2) failed to show any consistent relationship.

We then considered the possibility that the attitude of the investigators had changed – and that this was relevant to the

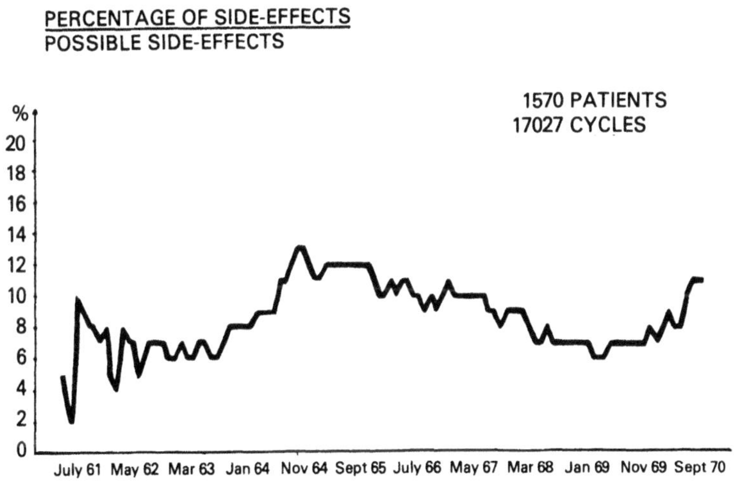

Figure 1 Incidence of side-effects

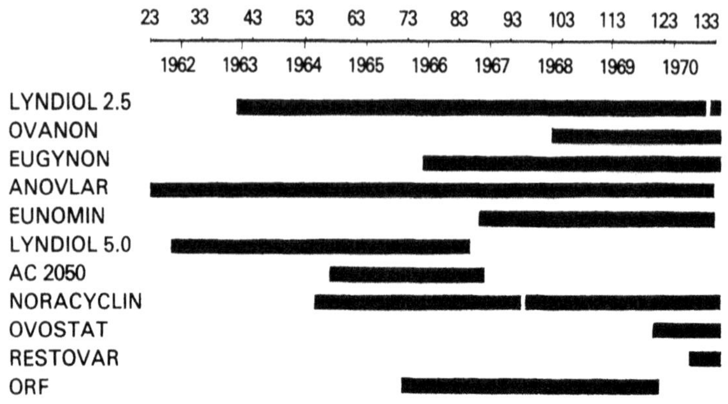

Figure 2 Distribution of oral contraceptive preparations during the period studied

reported incidence of side-effects. In the beginning we were sceptical about their efficacy and necessity, but later we had complete trust in them and were convinced they were one of the cornerstones of contraception. Significantly, the rate of side-effects reported was in inverse proportion to this change of attitude.

Previously (Figures 3 and 4), contraception had posed serious problems in our country, especially in central Switzerland, since the methods mainly practiced were the coitus interruptus and Knaus–Ogino methods – often as a bad combination (namely as alternatives). In the course of further clarification, we ascertained the number of reports about oral contraception that appeared in the mass media read in central Switzerland and we related these to the rate of side-effects reported (Figure 5). We gained the definite impression that every article in the mass media which referred to the side-effects of oral contraceptives and listed possible symptoms gave rise to a new increase in the incidence of their side-effects.

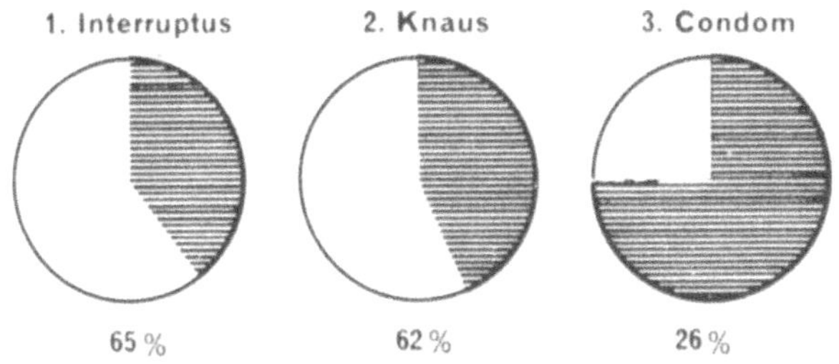

Figure 3 Most frequent contraceptive method (mostly in combination) in Switzerland

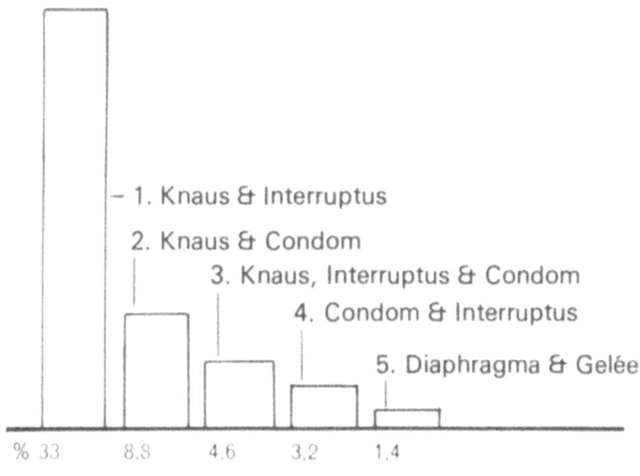

Figure 4 Most frequent combination of contraceptive method in Switzerland

In addition, we related the time when the special warnings of new side-effects were published in the specialist literature (and partly in the mass media) with the side-effects rate. There were three reports on the increased *incidence of thrombosis* (Figure 6); the last of which was launched on a big scale in the mass media but without a clear-cut sequel in the side-effects rate. We observed a distinct increase in the side-effects rate (Figure 7) after reports on the occurrence of an increased incidence of *mammary carcinoma* (in beagles) when progestogens alone were administered, even

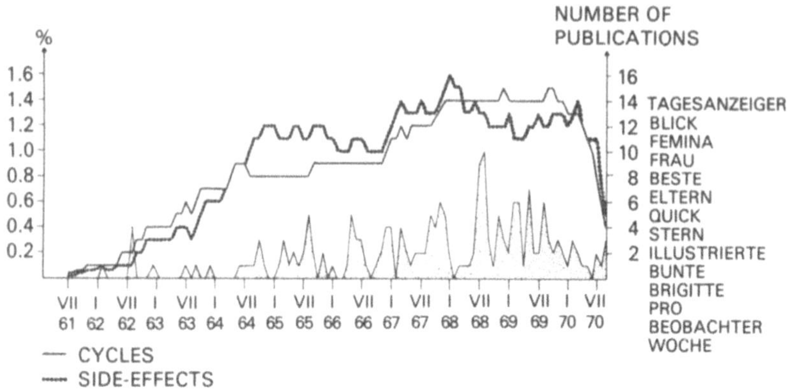

Figure 5 Distribution of cycles, frequency of side-effects and number of publications

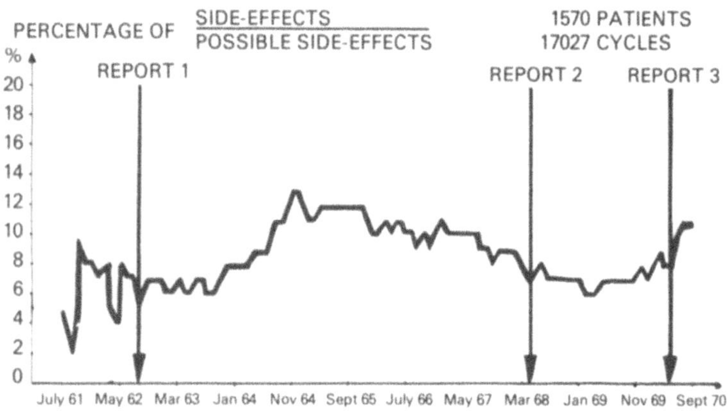

Figure 6 Percentages of side-effects reports concerning thrombosis

though they used unphysiologically high doses amounting to a multiple of those present in ovulation inhibitors. This reaction was probably accentuated by a broadcast appeal for women to consult their doctors. Five preparations were immediately withdrawn from the market.

Another, as far as we are concerned, potentially negative report went around the world when the papal encyclical '*Humanae Vitae*' (Abb. 8) appeared. In this encyclical, ovulation inhibitors were described as an unnatural method of fertility

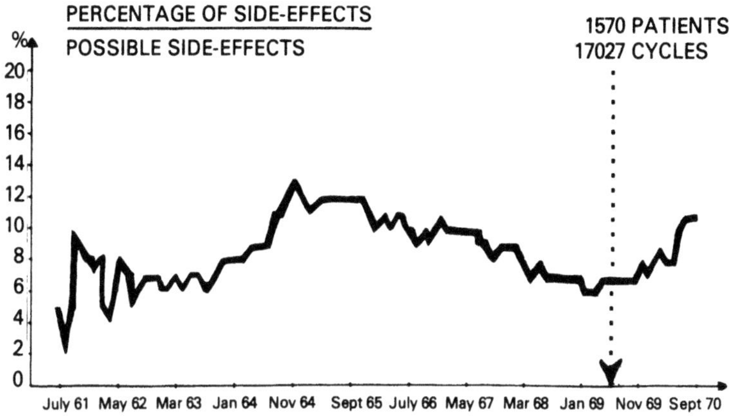

Figure 7 Incidence of side-effects following reports concerning beagle dogs

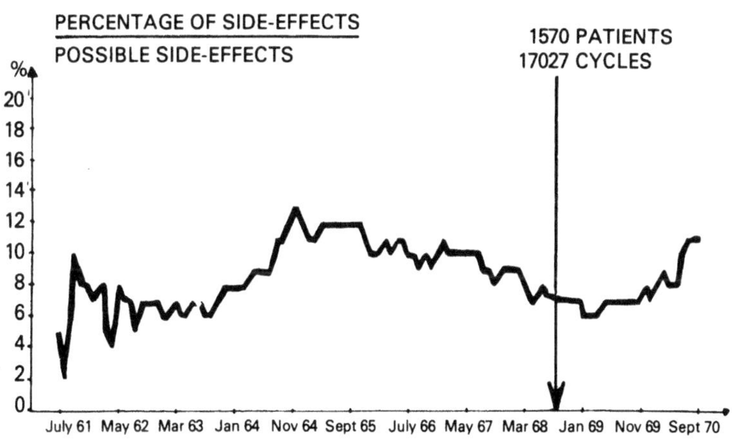

Figure 8 Incidence of side-effects following publication of the papal encyclical *Humanae Vitae*

control which was forbidden to Roman Catholics. This event was not associated with an increase in side-effects but rather with a decrease (see Figure 8). In time, however, Roman Catholics came to represent about 80% of my patients.

Further analysis of our patient population reveals that only 1% of Roman Catholics abandoned ovulation inhibitors on account of the encyclical. Since we know our patients, we can also observe that the ones who stopped taking ovulation inhibitors were not practising Roman Catholics, but rather women who are easy to influence (e.g., those who also follow the latest fashion). Such women are also said to be externally motivated.

Since about April or May 1975 we have been exposed to a number of negative reports on ovulation inhibitors, both in specialist journals and in the popular press. The first person to refer to 'pill tiredness' was Professor J. Zander, Munich, Senior Physician of the First Gynaecological Clinic, University of Munich, and a world-famous endocrinologist. He was addressing the Congress of the Austrian Society for Family Planning in Igls on May 2, 1975 and reported a number of patients who did not want to continue on the pill. Consequently, since this Congress was also attended by journalists, even reputable German magazines printed mainly negative reports on the pill (for example *Spiegel*, Figure 9, the magazine *Eltern*: Warum so viele Frauen die Pille nicht (mehr) nehmen wollen and the broadcasting station 'Rias Berlin'). These reports were repeated on Swiss radio under the title: 'The pill: hopes, experiences, disappointments'. The reports were based not only on personal experiences but also on information supplied by the Royal College of General Practitioners, which gave more weight to this theme.

All these reports were repeated and emphasized in other mass media, (inter alia *Playgirl*: The Dangers of Oral Contraception). Whereas in the first 10–15 years the reports published in the mass media tended to exaggerate the positive aspects of ovulation inhibitors, the reports appearing now are almost exclusively negative. This trend is not only apparent in Switzerland but also in Austria and Germany – and, a little later, in the United States. As a result, the President of the American Society of Gynecologists, H. L. Stone, as well as R. L. Miller, worried by this trend, attacked these reports verbally at the Congress of the Society in 1980, and in writing: 'The extra-ordinary zeal with which investigators have researched the pill has no precedent in medicine. They have found very little good in it and have brayed at the top of their lungs vis-à-vis media about all the possible problems in a manner some of us find quite offensive'[1] Further comments have underlined these observations:

THE BIG THREE 'P'S:

PROMISCUITY
PERMISSIVENESS
PILLS

ENCOURAGE VENEREAL DISEASES

Figure 9

'Both of the monetary support and the ego satisfaction, radio, television, and newspapers are used to spread the word. The patient hears it on the radio or reads it in the daily paper. Our journal will arrive some days later. We have, as one colleague in New York puts it, trial by media'[2]

'The bandwagon syndrome is associated with early acceptance of unimproved or popular ideas which are then disproved and abandoned only to be replaced by another fad'[2].

'Young women are fleeing the pill in large numbers and this portends ill for the future. Who wishes to return to the enormous numbers of unwanted pregnancies of the past with all the problems associated with them?'[1]

'The anti-pill flak should be turned down a bit because the alternative to a near perfect, effective contraceptive is usually pregnancy, which is not free from risk as we all know perfectly well, and this ought to be factored into the equation much more so than it presently is'[1].

'Lastly we emphasize that many girls and women of today are disturbed by the controversial discussion by the mass media relative to the contraceptive methods and they are partly misinformed. Here doctors can intervene by instructions'[3].

This world-wide campaign against oral contraceptives is a challenge for us doctors. If we do nothing the number of unwanted pregnancies will increase.

Our task is not only to clarify the real danger of the alternatives to oral contraception in papers and speeches for doctors but 'we must read what is being written in non-medical sources, especially bio-ethical articles and magazines for women. In this way we can get a better sense of the concerns of women regarding their health'[4].

References

1. Miller, R. L. (1980). For academica. *Am. J. Obstet. Gynecol.*, **137**, Nr. 6, S., 635
2. Stone, M. L. (1980). *Am. J. Obstet. Gynecol.*, **137**, Nr. 3, S., 309
3. Thormann, K. *et al.* (1982). Von Liebe träumen und an Kontrazeption denken, Therapeutische Umschau.
4. Nettles, J. B. (1980). *Am. J. Obstet. Gynecol.*, **137**, Nr. 3, S., 277

Chapter 3

Absence of correlation between oral contraceptive usage and ischemic heart disease

R. A. Wiseman

INTRODUCTION

The usage of oral contraceptives in the United Kingdom, as reflected by sales, rose from zero at their introduction in 1961 to 45 million packs at their peak in 1976, fell to 36 million in 1979, but rose again to 37 million packs in 1980.

Although many epidemiological studies have claimed an increased risk rate from overall circulatory mortality for oral contraceptive users[1-3], not only have the methods used been questioned[4] but others have been unable to find the increase in mortality rates for women of reproductive age that should have arisen if the claimed increased risk had actually occurred[5,6]. One recent publication showed that during the period when oral contraceptive usage rose in the United Kingdom, death rates from overall circulatory disease in women of reproductive age, far from increasing, actually fell steadily[7].

Similarly, for ischemic heart disease (IHD), although a number of epidemiological studies[1,2,8-11] have claimed an increased mortality and morbidity risk for oral contraceptive users as compared to non-users, usually of the order four to fivefold, there was no increase in notified mortality in the UK[7] or in Australia[12] nor of arterial disease in Sweden[13].

However, even though the recent publication from the Royal College of General Practitioners[14] stated that the main risk is for smokers, the authors still reported an increased cardiovascular mortality for oral contraceptive users. Moreover, despite their conclusion that increased duration of pill use is not associated with increased risk, they differentiated between women in different age groups, stating that the excess risk was largely concentrated in those aged 35 years or more. Because of this, it has been suggested[15,16] that examination of trends in mortality rates should be focused on that age group. It has been shown[17] that overall circulatory disease fell steadily even in this age group allegedly at risk, but it was thought that it would be worthwhile to examine IHD mortality rates in detail, not only for women of all reproductive age but particularly for those aged 35–44 years.

DATA SOURCES AND RESULTS

IHD mortality rates are derived from the Registrar General's Statistical Reviews England and Wales (1968–1973)[18] and Office of Population Censuses and Surveys Series DH2 (1974–1980)[19]. Classification of IHD (ICD numbers 410–414) differed before 1968 so continuity of comparison is not possible.

Table 1 IHD mortality rates, per million population

Year	*Female deaths by age* (y)				*Male deaths* (y)
	15–24	25–34	35–44	45–54	35–44
1968	2	15	107	419	647
1969	1	11	109	440	601
1970	1	8	101	419	657
1971	1	12	94	458	672
1972	2	13	106	524	664
1973	1	13	106	519	642
1974	1	9	110	512	647
1975	1	14	105	506	606
1976	1	12	110	510	588
1977	2	14	97	499	595
1978	1	14	103	520	616
1979	1	15	90	531	551
1980	1	14	85	458	543

The results are given in Table 1, from which it is seen that the rates for women of 15–24 years and 25–34 years have remained stable whilst those for women of 35–44 years have declined by 20%.

Table 2 Total pack sales of oral contraceptives in the United Kingdom

Year	*Sales*
1961	Conovid introduced
1964	3 750 000
1965	6 500 000
1966	8 350 000
1967	11 500 000
1968	14 150 000
1969	17 800 000
1970	18 100 000
1971	21 700 000
1972	26 000 000
1973	31 500 000
1974	36 000 000
1975	44 500 000
1976	45 100 000
1977	43 000 000
1978	38 650 000
1979	36 400 000
1980	37 100 000

Total pack sales of all oral contraceptives in the United Kingdom for the years 1961–1980 inclusive, obtained through the kindness of oral contraceptive manufacturers, are presented in Table 2. Both sets of data are shown graphically in Figure 1.

DISCUSSION

If the claimed causal association between oral contraceptive usage and IHD mortality is correct, then the stability of reported IHD mortality rates for women of 15–34 years and the decrease of 20% between the years 1968–1980 for women of 35–44 years is surprising in view of the increase in usage of oral contraceptives from 14 million packs in 1968 to the peak of 45 million in 1976.

It is important to determine whether some other relevant factor, acting to an extent equal to that alleged for oral contraceptives but in an opposite direction (i.e. a counteracting variable) has affected the mortality trend for women of 35–44 years and can therefore account for the decline in rates. Three possible counteracting variables – decreased ascertainment, decreased usage and decreased relative risk – need to be considered.

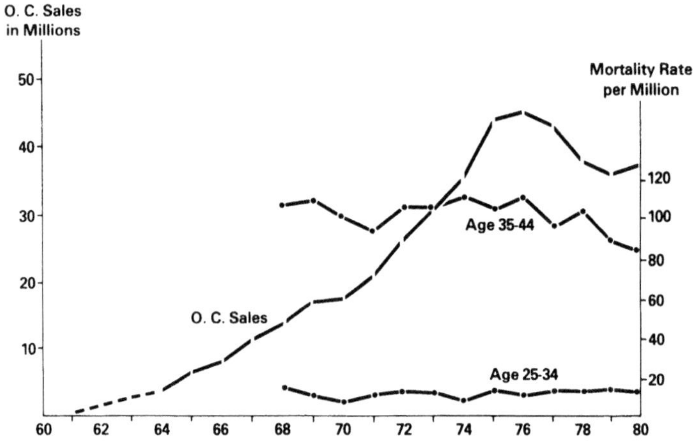

Figure 1 Oral contraceptive usage in the UK 1961–1980 and IHD mortality rates in females per 1 000 000 population 1968–1980

Decreased ascertainment

The decrease in mortality rates might be due to a decreased ascertainment exactly balancing a (true) increased incidence, but I judge this to be unlikely. Although there may be doubts about the accuracy and consistency of diagnoses entered into death certificates, I believe that every fatality due or suspected to be due to IHD in women of reproductive age in the UK is thoroughly investigated. Indeed, it is probable that when the diagnosis was in doubt IHD has been entered as the cause of death on death certificates of oral contraceptive users more readily than non-users due to the publicity associating this alleged side-effect with pill use, and thus there is likely to be a bias towards *increased* ascertainment. In addition, it is difficult to postulate a plausible reason why the (hypothesized) decreased ascertainment in 35–44 year-old women should coexist with an increase of 9% in notification rate for 45–54 year-old women, who, because they are generally beyond reproductive years, are not allegedly at risk from oral contraceptives and in whom therefore ascertainment and notification are likely to be less rigorous.

Decreased usage

It might be hypothesized that the decrease between 1968 and 1980 of IHD mortality rates in 35–44 year-old women is accounted for by a reduction in the absolute numbers of oral contraceptive users of that age group, despite the increase in total oral contraceptive usage for all age groups. However, available data do not confirm this: on the contrary, they show that the absolute numbers of oral contraceptive users of 35–44 years more than doubled. In 1968 there was a total population of 1.1 million of oral contraceptive users (calculated from the 14.1 million oral contraceptive packs sold) of whom 17.8% were aged 35–44 years, according to the RCGP Report[20] of 1974, i.e. 196 000. In 1976 there were 2.75 million women in the 35–44 year age group, in which it was reported[21] that oral contraceptive usage was 15%, i.e. 412 000 oral contraceptive users. Yet between these two years (1968 and 1976) the IHD mortality rates for this group of women altered hardly at all.

Moreover, any hypothesis concerning usage has also to explain the stable rates in the group of 25–34 year-old women, in which there has been a marked increase in oral contraceptive usage (both in absolute numbers and in percentage) and in which, according to the RCGP[14] and other studies[11], a relative risk of between 1.6 and 3.6 exists.

Decreased relative risk

It might be suggested that, although the number of users has increased for women aged 35–44 years, the relative risk over time has also changed, perhaps by a reduction in risk parallel to the reduction in estrogen content of oral contraceptives over the period under examination. It might be expected therefore that later studies would give lower relative risks – but this is not the case, as seen, for example, by the relative risks reported from the RCGP Study[14] (patient entry 1968–1969) and the higher ones from Boston Collaborative Drug Program[8] (patient entry 1975).

Thus, the possible counteracting variables considered above are unlikely to account for the falling IHD mortality rates in 35–44 year-old women between 1968 and 1980. Although the possibility of a further variable which might have kept the mortality rates artificially elevated cannot be totally rejected, there is no evidence in favor of that possibility and three sets of data which indicate that it is highly unlikely. First, although mortality rates for men of 35–44 years have fluctuated in individual years, over the period as a whole they declined by 12% (from a mean number of deaths per million of 624 for 1968/69 to a mean of 547 for 1979/80). Secondly, as we have seen, IHD mortality rates in 45–54 year-old women have increased. Thirdly, mortality rates in women of 35–44 years were almost identical in years (1969, 1974 and 1976) when oral contraceptive sales were widely different. If oral contraceptives are causally responsible for IHD it is reasonable to expect that the mortality rates in those allegedly at risk (women of 35–44 years) should not have decreased more steeply than those in men of comparable age, or should at least have increased to a greater degree than women who do not take oral contraceptives, and, in addition, have been different in years of different oral contraceptive usage. Yet none of these have occurred.

In conclusion, during the years 1968–1980 when oral contraceptive usage in the UK was increasing rapidly, IHD mortality rates in women of reproductive age either remained stable or, for those of 35–44 years, who are allegedly most at risk, declined. The absence of a positive correlation between oral contraceptive usage and IHD mortality rates, with no evidence in favor of and some against the existence of a counteracting variable, strongly suggests that there is no causal relationship between the two.

Thus, these results are opposed to the conclusions of a number of epidemiological studies which have claimed an increased IHD risk rate for all women of reproductive age who use oral contraceptives as compared to non-users, and specifically contradict the suggestion that such increased risk is found in 35–44 year-old women.

SUMMARY

Oral contraceptive usage, and IHD mortality rates for all women of reproductive age and specifically for those aged 35–44 years have been examined for the years 1968–1980 in the United Kingdom. These data show:

(1) Oral contraceptive usage increased from 14.1 million packs in 1968, to 45.1 million in 1976, decreasing to 37.1 million in 1980.

(2) IHD mortality rates for women of reproductive age of 15–34 years were remarkably stable: for those aged 35–44 years the rate fell gradually by 20% between 1968 and 1980.

The absence of a positive correlation between these two sets of data is difficult to explain if a causal relationship exists between them, as claimed by some epidemiological studies.

Possible counteracting variables – such as decreased ascertainment or decreased usage by women of 35–44 years, or decreased relative risk over the time period – which might account for this paradoxical result, are examined but discarded as being unlikely. Evidence from other mortality data, which suggests that a counteracting variable does not exist, is presented.

Thus the data on IHD mortality rates in the UK, showing an absence of positive correlation with oral contraceptive usage, are opposed to the conclusions of epidemiological studies claiming an increased risk of IHD mortality due to oral contraceptives, and specifically contradict the claim that such increased risk is found in 35–44 year-old oral contraceptive users.

Acknowledgement

I would like to thank Miss Sue Claughton and Mrs Jill Harwood for assistance in the preparation of this paper.

References

1. Royal College of General Practitioners' Oral Contraceptive Study (1977). Mortality among oral contraceptive users. *Lancet*, **2**, 727
2. Vessey, M. P., McPherson, K. and Johnson, B. (1977). Mortality among women participating in the Oxford Family Planning Association contraceptive study. *Lancet*, **2**, 731
3. Petitti, D. B., Wingerd, J., Pellegrin, F. and Ramcharan, S. (1979). Risk of vascular disease in women: smoking, oral contraceptives, non-contra-

ceptive estrogens and other factors. *J. Am. Med. Assoc.*, **242**, 1150
4. Horwitz, R. I. and Feinstein, A. R. (1979). Methodological standards and contradictory results in case-control research. *Am. J. Med.*, **66**, 556
5. Tietze, C. (1979). The pill and mortality from cardiovascular disease: another look. *Fam. Plann. Perspect.*, **11**, 80
6. Belsey, M. A., Russell, Y. and Kinnear, K. (1979). Cardiovascular disease and oral contraceptives: a reappraisal of vital statistics data. *Fam. Plann. Perspect.*, **11**, 84
7. Wiseman, R. A. and MacRae, K. D. (1981). Oral contraceptives and the decline in mortality from circulatory disease. *Fertil. Steril.*, **35**, 277
8. Jick, H., Dinan, B. and Rothman, K. J. (1978). Oral contraceptives and non-fatal myocardial infarction. *J. Am. Med. Assoc.*, **239**, 1403
9. Shapiro, S., Rosenbert, L., Slone, D., Kaufman, D. W., Stolley, P. D. and Miettinen, O. S. (1979). Oral contraception in relation to myocardial infarction. *Lancet*, **1**, 743
10. Hennekens, C. H., Evans, D. and Peto, R. (1979). Oral contraceptive use, cigarette smoking and myocardial infarction. *Br. J. Fam. Plann.*, **5**, 66
11. Slone, D., Shapiro, S., Kaufman, D. W., Rosenberg, L., Miettinen, O. S. and Stolley, P. D. (1981). Risk of myocardial infarction in relation to current and discontinued use of oral contraceptives. *N. Engl. J. Med.*, **305**, 420
12. Shearman, R. P. (1981). Oral contraceptives: where are the excess deaths? *Med. J. Aust.*, **1**, 698
13. Bottiger, L. E., Boman, G., Eklund, G. and Westerholm, B. (1980). Oral contraceptives and thromboembolic disease: effects of lowering oestrogen content. *Lancet*, **1**, 1097
14. Royal College of General Practitioners' Oral Contraception Study (1981). Further analyses of mortality in oral contraceptive users. *Lancet*, **1**, 541
15. Layde, P. M., Rubin, R. M. and Ory, H. W. (1981). Oral contraceptives and circulatory disease. *Fertil. Steril.*, **36**, 412
16. Vessey, M. P. and Mann, J. I. (1981). Oral contraceptives and circulatory disease. *Fertil. Steril.*, **36**, 413
17. Wiseman, R. A. and MacRae, K. D. (1981). Oral contraceptives and circulatory disease. *Fertil. Steril.*, **36**, 414
18. Registrar General's Statistical Review of England and Wales for years 1968–1973. (1970–1975). Part I (Table 17) and Part II (Table A2). (London: Her Majesty's Stationery Office)
19. Office of Population Censuses and Surveys (1976–1980). Series DH2 Mortality Statistics (Cause) for years 1974–1980, Table 3 (London: Her Majesty's Stationery Office)
20. Royal College of General Practitioners' Oral Contraception Study (1974). *Oral contraceptives and health.* Chap. 8, Table 2.1. (London: Pitman Medical)
21. Dunnell, K. (1979). *Office of Population Censuses and Surveys: Family Formation 1976.* Chap. 41. (London: Her Majesty's Stationery Office)

Chapter 4

Australian experiences with hormonal contraception over two decades

J. H. Evans

SUMMARY

In the early 1960s the highest rates of oral contraceptive usage were in Australia and New Zealand, followed by the USA and Canada. By 1973 these countries had been joined by the Netherlands and West Germany.

Audits have clearly revealed the effects of the various medical reports warning about the possible hazards of hormonal contraception. The principal hazards publicized in 1969 and 1970 resulted in discontinuation of usage in over 15% of Australian women.

Despite further medical misgivings and adverse media coverage in 1977, there has been continuing usage and popularity of hormonal contraception and, recently, evidence of an upturn in use.

Virtually all the data reporting side-effects of hormonal contraception comes from developed countries and from studies carried out at a time when preparations contained high doses of both estrogen and progestogen. The introduction of lower dosage and lower risk formulations underlines the need to identify and inform the woman at risk.

THE STUDY

After two decades of use, oral contraceptives remain the most popular reversible form of contraception in the world today.

Throughout the world at least 150 million women have used oral contraceptives since they first became available, and at present over 60 million women are using this highly effective form of contraception. Usage has indeed been influenced over the years by medical misgivings about some aspects of the use of steroidal contraception and by media coverage, usually expressed in most dramatic terms. Despite this, usage rates for women aged 15–44 y range up to 40% in developed countries and are increasing rapidly in the developing countries (Figure 1).

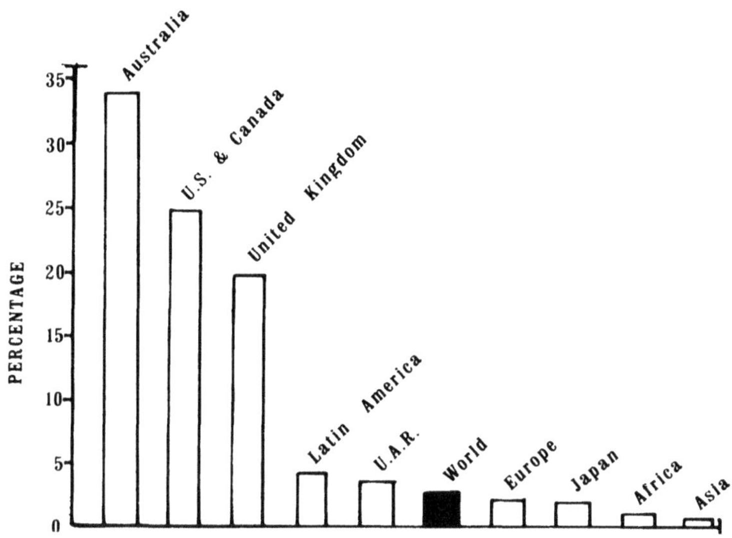

Figure 1 Percentage of married women of childbearing age (15–44 y) using oral contraceptives 1968

Combined oral contraceptives consisting of an estrogen and progestogen component first became available in Australia in early 1961 and the Australian woman readily accepted their usage. By 1968 almost 35% of married women of childbearing age in Australia were using the pill[1]. This percentage was greater than that in either the USA and Canada or the United Kingdom. By 1970, more than 20% of Australian women of reproductive age were supplied with oral contraceptives through commercial channels. As the content of estrogen and progestogen changed, acceptance of hormonal contraception steadily increased and by 1975 one Australian woman in three between the age of 15 and 44 years was purchasing oral contraceptives regularly. The only country exceeding this incidence was the Netherlands (Table 1, Figure 2).

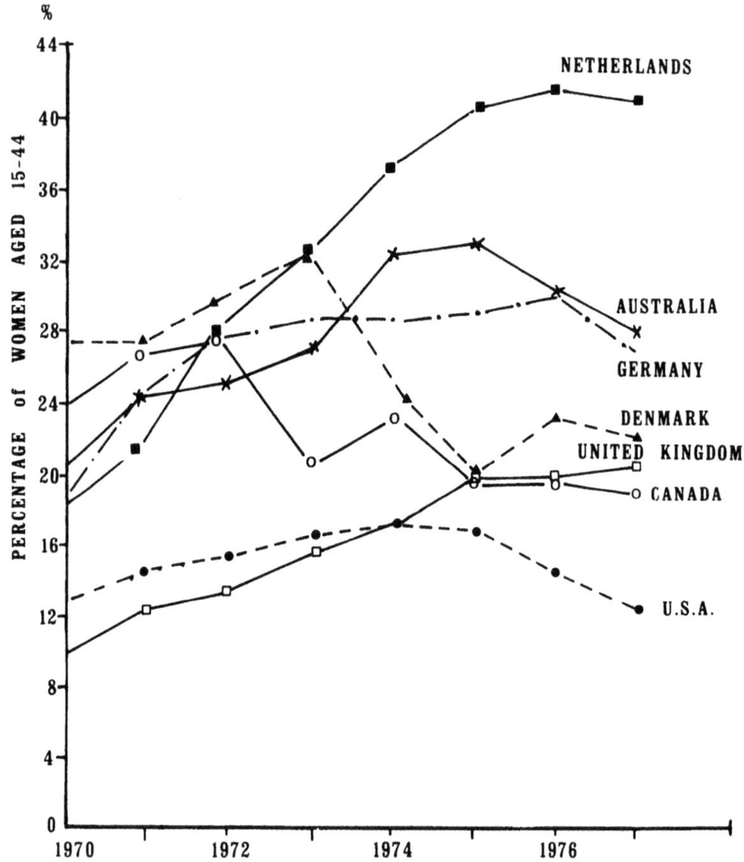

Figure 2 Minimum percentage of women aged 15–44 supplied with oral contraceptives through commercial channels in some developed countries 1970–1977

Table 1 Minimum percentage of women aged 15–44 supplied with oral contraceptives through commercial channels 1970–1977

	1970	1971	1972	1973	1974	1975	1976	1977
Australia	20.2	24.2	25.6	27.2	32.5	33.4	30.3	28.0
Canada	23.9	26.4	27.7	21.7	23.4	19.4	19.6	18.7
Denmark	27.5	27.6	29.9	32.1	24.9	20.3	23.2	22.2
German Federal Republic	18.9	24.4	27.6	28.7	28.6	29.3	30.0	26.8
The Netherlands	18.6	21.8	28.1	32.8	37.7	40.5	41.2	40.8
United Kingdom	9.9	12.1	13.4	15.5	16.9	19.8	19.8	20.3
United States	12.7	14.4	15.4	16.7	17.1	16.8	14.5	12.2

Audits have clearly revealed the effects of the various medical reports warning about the possible hazards of oral contraception. The principal hazards publicized in 1969 and 1970 of an increased risk of thromboembolism and stroke in contraceptive users resulted in a sudden fall of contraceptive pill sales throughout Australia by 15% (Pharmaceutical Research Services of Australia, 1971). 53% of those women who ceased taking oral contraceptives stated that adverse publicity had influenced their decision and such adverse publicity at the time outnumbered favorable publicity by five to one[2]. Patients who had continued to use oral contraception were noted to be those keeping in close contact with family planning clinics and physicians.

Such an impact was not as evident in Europe and especially Germany. Within 2 years of this initial adverse publicity, when further evaluations put earlier warnings into a more reassuring perspective, and with the introduction of lower dosage formulations, usage once more increased.

In February 1973, oral contraceptives became available as a pharmaceutical benefit item and within 2 years one third of Australian women of reproductive age were using hormonal contraception (Table 2).

In 1977, a further temporary downward trend in sales was again noted, with the release of the report of circulatory system disease in association with oral contraceptive usage. However, as had been observed following the adverse publicity earlier in the decade, such a slump was to be temporary only and the total number of prescriptions written in Australia has once again slowly but steadily increased.

Table 2 Pharmaceutical benefits: oral contraceptives

Year	*Total prescriptions**
1973–1974	5 243 564
1974–1975	5 851 037
1975–1976	6 010 482
1976–1977	5 803 096
1977–1978	5 429 191
1978–1979	5 096 572
1979–1980	4 866 868
1980–1981	4 904 435

*6 months supply per prescription

Ever since the early 1970s, following the evidence linking hormonal contraception with an increased incidence of thrombosis, research has concentrated on lowering the doses of the steroids in the standard estrogen/progestogen combination preparation.

Initially it was believed to be more important to lower the dose of estrogen, as this had been shown to be the major steroid affecting blood factors linked with clot formation. During the late 1970s biochemical data and epidemiological studies commenced to incriminate the progestogen also as an etiological factor in certain unwanted side-effects, the relationship being noted with increasing dose and potency of the progestogen in the presence of constant estrogen dosage.

As a result, the recent formulations available contain the lowest possible doses of both synthetic steroids. That this is beneficial is commencing to emerge from population studies which show lower morbidity and mortality rates in the users of these lower dosage and therefore lower risk preparations.

With respect to the safety of hormonal contraception, the major cohort studies on either side of the Atlantic have indicated that the risks associated with their usage do not apply to all women equally. Circulatory system disease, for example, is more likely in the oral contraceptive user over the age of 35 years who smokes or has other factors predisposing to the development of circulatory disease.

Virtually all the data concerning these side-effects come from countries where circulatory disease and the factors predisposing to same are common. The findings in studies in Britain and the United States cannot automatically be applied to women in Australia or in the developing countries.

As the use of hormonal contraception enters its third decade, the trend is towards the lower dosage and lower risk preparation. Some of the initial fears associated with the use of the higher dose preparations – especially the adverse effects on subsequent fertility and on offspring conceived after its use – have eased with the efflux of time. At present there is no unequivocal evidence to indicate a relationship between the use of oral contraceptives and secondary amenorrhea subsequent to its use in those cases where the duration of the amenorrhea is greater than 6 months. Also unresolved is the question of carcinogenicity of sex steroids.

Whilst further clarification of the potential risks and of the possible benefits of hormonal contraception is awaited, present evidence suggests that the safer preparations are those which contain lower dosages of steroids. Preparations containing less than 50 μg of estrogen were introduced into Australia in 1975 and have proven most satisfactory although, as anticipated, with the reduction in dosage there has been an increased incidence of breakthrough bleeding.

Likewise, erratic bleeding patterns have been encountered in women on the progestogen only preparations, which, being estrogen-free and containing very low doses of progestogens, are associated with the lowest risks of all hormonal contraceptives.

The triphasic preparations have been available in Australia

since August 1981, and early studies pertinent to cycle control with their use are extremely promising (Table 3).

Table 3 Australia: oral contraceptives

Combination
19 formulations
44 packagings
Progestogen only
2 formulations
4 packagings

Available in Australia at present are 48 different oral contraceptives. If one excludes the progestogen only pills, the remaining 44 products contain 19 different combinations of estrogens and progestogens. The efficacy of the preparations remains unchanged, reliable contraception being maintained. The lowering of dosage has reduced the hazards of the oral contraceptive, enabling some women at risk the continued use of effective contraception.

The greatest potential in research into contraception continues to be to find methods which, whilst effective, are free of systemic effects. In the meantime, both doctors and users must attempt to identify those who are at risk and, dependent upon the benefit/risk analysis for that individual, prescribe accordingly. Careful counselling and supervision are required for all women with risk factors and the prescriber must be ever alert for the development of new risk factors.

References

1. Peel, J. and Potts, M. (1969). *Text Book of Contraceptive Practice.* p. 127. (Cambridge: Cambridge University Press)
2. Bertuch, G. and Leeton, J. (1971). The effect of publicity on oral contraceptive practice. *Med. J. Aust.*, **2**, 1067

Discussion

Question Dr Diczfalusy, as you took the male contraceptive pill as your 'model' does gossypol meet the criteria you described for use in human beings?

Dr Diczfalusy Gossypol has only been used in 8006 patients so far. It is not yet ready for clinical testing according to the criteria I described.

Question Your investigation deals only with mortality rates. Is it not possible there has been an increase in morbidity rates of ischemic heart disease as a consequence of pill use, but mortality rates have decreased because of better medical care?

Dr Wiseman If there had been better medical care, it should have affected to an equal degree males of comparable age and older women, yet their mortality rates have differed from each other and from those of 35–44 year-old women. I do not think therefore that it is reasonable to hypothesize that better medical care can account for trends in mortality rates which have gone in opposite directions in different age- and sex-groups. Whether or not it has affected morbidity rates, I cannot say.

In any event, I am much more suspicious about morbidity rates (about which there are no data) than mortality rates because of the difficulties of ensuring a precise diagnosis. I feel a diagnosis in the United Kingdom is likely to be more accurate after a young woman on an oral contraceptive has died and a postmortem has been carried out than when a young woman is admitted to hospital with chest pains and recovery occurs.

Finally, of course, many of the epidemiological studies whose conclusions I have questioned claim an increased relative risk due to oral contraceptives of mortality, not morbidity, and this is the problem which I have addressed.

Question Have you taken into account whether 45–54-year-old women, whose mortality rates for ischemic heart disease have risen, were on oral contraceptives for ten or more years, say from the age of 25 onwards?

Dr Wiseman I have no data on which of these women were or were not on oral contraceptives. However, I feel that such a long-term effect is unlikely, because if it had occurred I would have expected at least some effect in younger women also, i.e. between 35–44 years, many of whom have also been on oral contraceptives for 10 years or more yet whose IHD rates have fallen. Moreover, such a speculation contradicts the results of a number of epidemiological studies which have not claimed any increased risk with increasing duration of contraceptive use.

Section II

Clinical Experiences with the New Triphasic Oral Contraceptive

Moderator: A. A. Haspels

Chapter 5

Clinical performance of a triphasic administration of ethinyl estradiol and levonorgestrel in comparison with the 30 + 150 μg fixed-dose regime

G. Zador

SUMMARY

In order to assess the overall tolerance of a new triphasic oral contraceptive containing ethinyl estradiol and levonorgestrel in comparison with a well-known low-dose pill containing the same hormones, 489 women were assigned at random to one of these two preparations. The study was planned to run over a period of 6 consecutive months and the case report forms were designed in a fashion to permit comparable evaluation of the two formulations with regard to their overall reliability and clinical performance, mainly in terms of cycle control.

The 489 volunteers, who were uniformly selected on the basis of their meeting the requirements for the prescription of oral contraceptives in accordance with established medical practice, completed 2777 cycles. No pregnancy occurred during the observation period. Approximately 90% of the patients completed the six months treatment period. Withdrawal bleeding failed to occur in only 0.9% of the total cycles in women taking the triphasic pill and in 2.3% of the total cycles in women using the fixed dose combination. During the course of treatment a continuous transition from longer and heavier menstruations to shorter and scantier ones was observed by the patients in both groups. Bleeding irregularities, such as spotting and/or breakthrough bleedings occurred more frequently on the

30/150 μg pill compared with the triphasic formulation (16% versus 10% of women). Altogether 9% of the women on each pill discontinued treatment for medical reasons, the most common of which was spotting.

From the present study it can be concluded that the new triphasic formulation seems to be just as safe as the well-known 30/150 μg pill, but it appears to be superior to the 30/150 μg pill in terms of a lower incidence of various bleeding irregularities.

INTRODUCTION

After two decades of use, oral contraceptives are the most widely used reversible method of contraception today, and there are now more than 60 million women throughout the world using this highly effective form of birth control[1]. The fact that hormonal contraception involves the prolonged use of potent drugs in healthy people means these preparations are some of the most carefully scrutinized drugs and coincidental medical problems and adverse effects have become a great concern of the medical profession. Initially research suggested that the estrogen component of the pill was responsible for morbidity related to the combination pill[2], but a recent report implicated the progestogen component as well[3]. In a continuous effort to minimize various metabolic changes by combined oral contraceptives that might lead to untoward effects it seems now also logical to bring about a substantial reduction in the progestogen component of the pill but without compromising efficacy and tolerance.

Based on earlier experience it is not likely that the levonorgestrel quantity, in combination with the low amount of 30 μg ethinyl estradiol, can be reduced beyond a critical 150 μg level when using a conventional fixed dose schedule throughout the cycle mainly because of expected poor cycle control. The development of a new triphasic administration of ethinyl estradiol and levonorgestrel was based on the assumption that mimicking the physiological fluctuation in the blood levels of estradiol-17β and progesterone, which are found during the normal menstrual cycles, may allow a further reduction in the total steroid content of the pill without compromising patient tolerance by poor cycle control.

The aim of the present study was to assess the tolerance, principally in terms of cycle control, of this triphasic combined oral contraceptive in a controlled, randomized comparative study with the well-established 30 μg ethinyl estradiol plus 150 μg levonorgestrel pill.

MATERIALS AND METHOD

The composition of the triphasic pill* is shown in Figure 1. During the first 6 days there are 30 μg ethinyl estradiol (EE_2) in

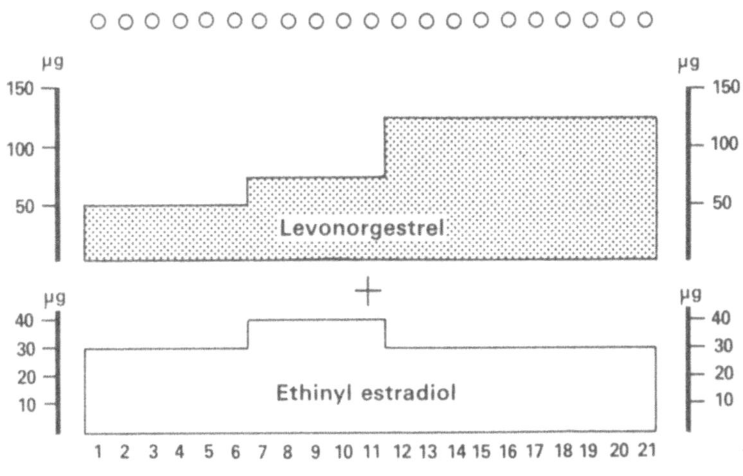

Figure 1 Composition of the triphasic combined oral contraceptive

*Triphasic pill: Triquilar[R], Trigynon[R], Logynon[R], Trionetta[R], Triagynon[R], Trikvilar[R]

combination with 50 μg levonorgestrel (LNg) and in the following 5 days 40 μg EE_2 with 75 μg LNg. Finally, over the last 10 days, 30 μg of EE_2 is combined with 125 μg LNg.

Altogether 489 women took part in this randomized multicenter study – 254 women in the triphasic group and 235 in the well-known fixed dose type combined oral contraceptive (30 μg EE_2/150 μg LNg)** group.

In terms of total hormone intake there is a slightly higher dose level of EE_2 per cycle in the triphasic pill (680 μg EE_2 per cycle) compared with 630 μg, but there is a substantial difference in the levonorgestrel levels, 1.9 mg per cycle (triphasic pill) compared with 3.15 mg per cycle.

Identical protocols suitable for computer analysis were used and there was no difference in the patient material with regard to age distribution, parity, or number of previous miscarriages. Generally, patients were selected on the basis of their meeting the requirements for the prescription of oral contraceptives in accordance with established medical practice. The purposes of the study were explained to the patients before enrolment and only those who gave their verbal consent and were prepared to participate for the entire 6 months duration of the trial were accepted.

Details concerning menstrual losses, intermenstrual bleeding or spotting and other encountered side-effects were recorded carefully by the women and noted on a chart given to them by the doctor.

Intermenstrual bleeding was classified as 'breakthrough bleeding' when the quantity of blood loss required the use of any sanitary protection, and as 'spotting' in all other cases including also slight brownish discharge. Detailed routine gynecological examinations including blood pressure and body weight, were performed prior to the trial. Follow-up visits were requested after 1, 3 and 6 months in order to report pertinent clinical

**30 μg EE_2/150 μg LNg: Microgynon[R] 30, Neovletta[R]

events and to record body weight and blood pressure.

The total patient material with respect to age and drug distribution is shown in Figure 2.

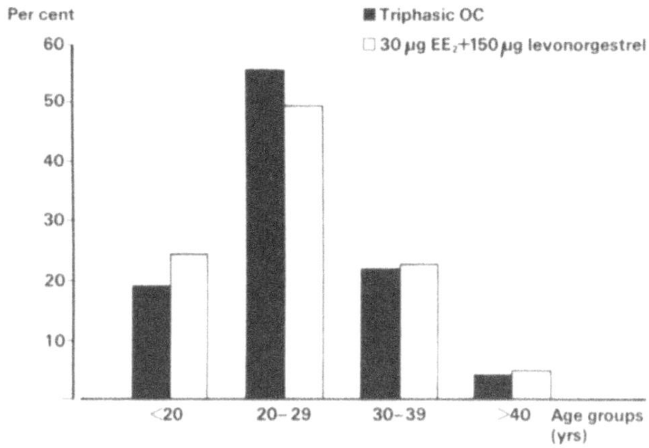

Figure 2 Age distribution of the 489 participants in the study – expressed as percentage of the total patient material

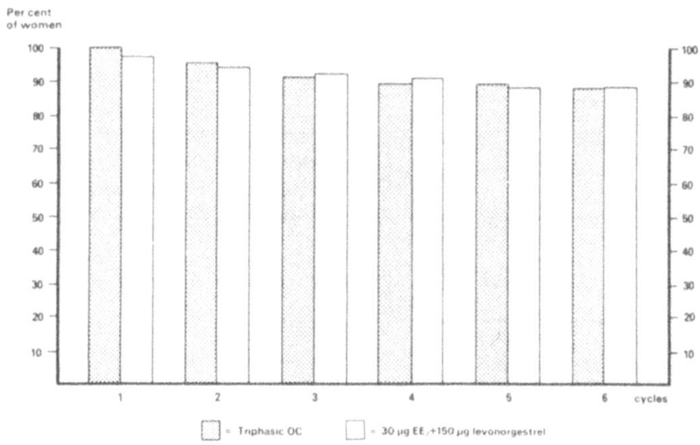

Figure 3 Percentage of women completing each cycle (n=254 for the triphasic oral contraceptive and 235 for the 30 µg EE_2/150 µg LNg pill)

RESULTS

The 489 women completed a total number of 2777 cycles. The percentage of women completing the six cycles is shown in Figure 3. On average, 90% of the subjects on both drugs completed the 6 months treatment period, which was regarded as sufficient time in which to study cycle control and bleeding irregularities, the two major purposes of this clinical trial.

Efficacy

No pregnancy occurred during the observation period.

Duration of menstruation

During the last cycle prior to the start of the study, most patients were having periods of approximately 5 days. During the course of treatment there was a continuous transition from longer menstruations to shorter ones in both groups (Table 1). It also appears from this Table that the reduction of the menstrual period was somewhat more pronounced in women taking the 30 μg EE_2/150 μg LNg pill.

Table 1 Duration of menstruation in days prior to and after 6 months of treatment (mean ± SD)

	Triphasic oral contraceptive	*30 μg EE_2 + 150 μg levonorgestrel*
Last untreated cycle	5.3 ± 0.9	5.0 ± 1.2
After the 6th treatment cycle	3.9 ± 0.8	3.2 ± 1.0

Intensity

The intensity of menstrual bleeding before and at different phases of treatment showed practically the same pattern (Figure

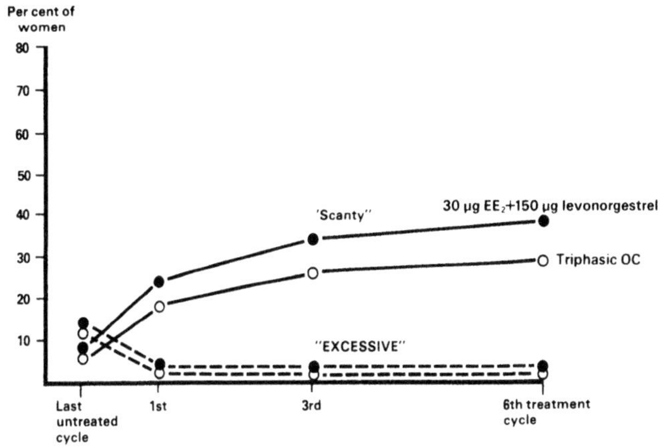

Figure 4 Intensity of menstrual flow before and at different phases of treatment

4). The amount of menstrual flow, defined by the participants as 'scanty', 'moderate' or 'excessive' was reduced during the course of treatment; approximately 15% of the women had reported 'excessive' menstrual bleeding prior to medication. This figure decreased right from the first treatment cycles to approximately 5%. 'Scanty' bleeding was reported in an ever increasing frequency by women taking both drugs, but the increase was more pronounced in women receiving 30 µg EE_2/150 µg LNg.

Withdrawal bleeding

The missed withdrawal bleeding calculated in relation to the total number of cycles showed that, among women taking the triphasic preparation, 13 cycles were followed by missed bleeding out of a total of 1440 (0.9%) while, on 30 µg EE_2/150 µg LNg, this occurred in 31 cycles out of a total of 1337 cycles (2.3%). This difference is statistically significant ($p<0.001$).

Intermenstrual bleeding/spotting

The percentage of women reporting intermenstrual bleeding/spotting before and during treatment revealed a very important difference between the two preparations. Among those allocated to the triphasic drug, 4.4% had reported intermenstrual bleeding before treatment, while on 30 μg EE_2/150 μg LNg, only 1.7% did so (Figure 5). Despite this, following the first and second cycles of treatment 10.3% of subjects using the triphasic pill reported spotting compared with 21.4% using 30 μg EE_2/150 μg LNg. With respect to breakthrough bleeding the corresponding figures were 4.6% for the triphasic pill and 7.2% for the fixed combination pill. In the third to sixth cycles the difference was not so pronounced but still slightly in favor of the triphasic preparation.

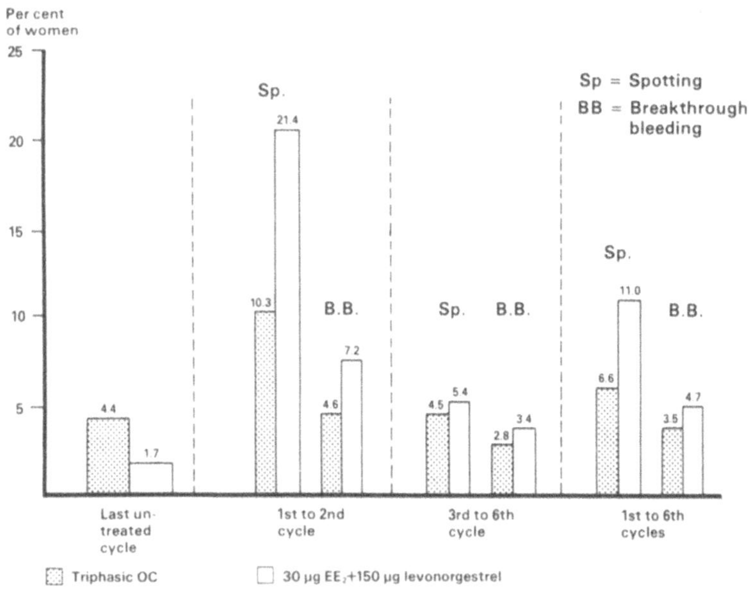

Figure 5 Percentage of women reporting intermenstrual bleeding/spotting before and during treatment

Body weight

The vast majority of women, approximately 85%, retained their pretreatment weight within a variation of ± 2 kg following the sixth treatment cycle.

Side-effects

Side-effects reported by the users were of the types commonly associated with oral contraceptive use and their significance to the types of treatment given was not possible to evaluate with certainty.

Blood pressure

No significant changes in blood pressure were recorded throughout the treatment period.

Patient withdrawal

A total of 72 out of 489 women, corresponding to 14.7% of the total entering the study, discontinued treatment before the stipulated time of 6 months. Of these, 44 (9%) discontinued for medical reasons, the most common of which was bleeding irregularities. The remaining 28 (5.7%) women discontinued for non-medical, i.e. personal reasons (Table 2). There was no significant difference between the two preparations with respect to the discontinuation rate.

Table 2 Reasons for discontinuing treatment

	Triphasic oral contraceptive	*30 µg EE_2/150 µg LNg*
Medical reasons	23 (9%)	21 (8.9%)
Personal reasons	13 (5.1%)	15 (6.3%)
Total number of women discontinuing treatment	36 (14.1%)	36 (15.2%)

DISCUSSION

Both oral contraceptives tested in the present trial were equally safe and effective as no pregnancies occurred.

Briggs[4] pointed out that the oral contraceptive of choice for the majority of women is a combination of ethinyl estradiol and norgestrel and that the lowest dose of each of these components compatible with maximum safety and patient acceptability should be used. The new triphasic pill represents a new generation of combined oral contraceptives in so far as it combines the advantages of a 30 μg ethinyl estradiol low-dose preparation with a substantial reduction of the total progestogen amount when compared with the 30 μg EE_2/150 μg LNg pill. The reduction of levonorgestrel is highly justified due to reports indicating that oral contraceptives containing progestogens of the 19-nortestosterone derivative type result in reduced HDL-lipoprotein concentration in the blood[5], a fact which might accelerate the development of atherosclerosis[6], and that the concentration of HDL-cholesterol, in general, decreases with increasing dose of progestogen.

The major aim of the present study was to carefully assess the overall tolerance principally in terms of cycle control, of a new triphasic administration of ethinyl estradiol plus levonorgestrel in comparison with the 30 μg EE_2/150 μg LNg pill.

The study has convincingly shown, that in spite of the considerably reduced levonorgestrel amount, the triphasic pill is clearly superior to the fixed dose preparation in terms of lower incidence of intermenstrual spotting and bleeding and a significantly lower incidence of missed withdrawal bleeding. Both these findings, which are visualized in Figure 6, are of great clinical importance because women often stop taking an oral contraceptive if they experience poor cycle control. Furthermore, missed periods usually cause patients unnecessary fear of being pregnant and in many unnecessary tests to rule out pregnancies.

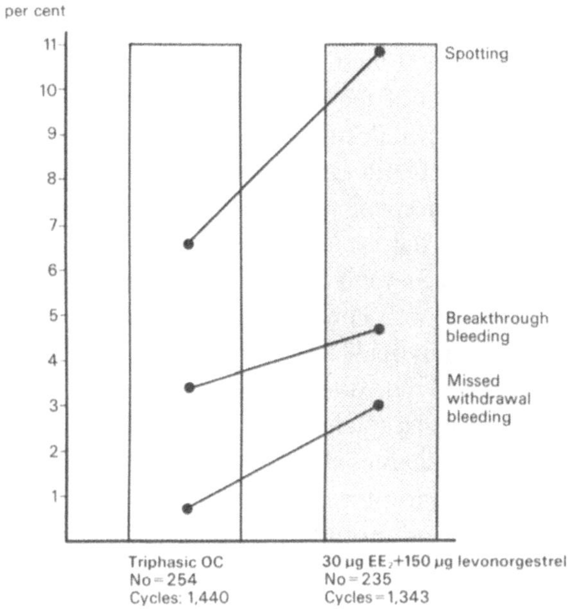

Figure 6 Comparison of bleeding irregularities encountered with the two pills. Expressed as percentage of women reporting such incidences throughout the six treatment cycles

Following the first and second cycles of treatment 10.3% of subjects using the triphasic pill reported spotting compared with 21.4% using 30 μg EE_2/150 μg LNg. These figures perhaps seem to be rather high, but in this study we made it very clear to the patients that they should report every incidence of bleeding, even the slightest, brownish discharge, because otherwise it would be difficult for them to differentiate and to determine what was and was not spotting.

In the present study not too much attention was paid to subjective side-effects related to oral contraceptive medication, because only 6 months treatment in a rather limited number of patients was considered too short a period to be worthwhile in trying to make far-reaching conclusions in this respect. Even when placebo is given, there are reported side-effects very similar to those found during oral contraceptive medication[7] and consequently we were mostly interested in cycle control.

The development of the presently tested new triphasic oral contraceptive clearly reflects the progress made over the years in reducing the dose of both estrogen and progestogen component of the pill[8]. The concept of mimicking sex steroid serum levels of the normal menstrual cycle has resulted in clearly improved cycle control when compared to other low-dose preparations. In addition, this new oral contraceptive causes only minimal, if any, deterioration in lipid[9] and carbohydrate metabolism[10].

In conclusion, the present study, in conformity with additional clinical data generated and presented elsewhere in this publication (Chapter 8), strongly indicates that the new triphasic oral contraceptive seems to be a very promising new generation of oral contraceptive. It should, however, be pointed out that owing to the very low hormone intake, appropriate counselling of potential users is essential to reduce the incidence of bleeding problems and consequently the discontinuation rate, and, what is maybe even more important, the risk of unwanted pregnancies.

References

1. Kleinman, R. L. (ed.) (1981). *IPPF Medical Bulletin* **15**, 6
2. Speroff, L., Glass, R. H. and Kase, N. G. (1968). *Clinical Gynecologic Endocrinology and Infertility*. p. 300. (Baltimore: Williams and Wilkins)
3. Royal College of General Practitioners Oral Contraceptive Study (1977). Effect of hypertension and benign breast disease of progestogen component in combined oral contraceptives. *Lancet*, **1**, 624
4. Briggs, M. H. (1975). Effects of oral progestogens on estrogen induced changes in plasma proteins. *J. Reprod. Med.*, **15**, 100
5. Bradley, D. D., Wingerd, J., Petitti, D. B., Kraus, R. M. and Ramcharan, S. (1978). Serum high density lipoprotein cholesterol in women using oral contraceptives, estrogens and progestins. *N. Engl. J. Med.*, **299**, 17
6. Jenkins, P. J., Harper, R. W. and Nestel, P. J. (1978). Severity of coronary atherosclerosis related to lipoprotein concentration. *Br. Med. J.*, **2**, 388

7. Goldzieher, J. W., Moses, L. E., Averkin, E., Scheel, C. and Taber, B. Z. (1971). A placebo controlled double-blind crossover investigation of the side-effects attributed to oral contraception. *Fertil. Steril.*, **22**, 609
8. Lachnit-Fixson, U. (1980). The rationale for a new triphasic contraceptive. In Greenblatt, R. B. (ed.) *The Development of a New Triphasic Oral Contraceptive.* pp. 23–29. (Lancaster: MTP Press)
9. Larsson-Cohn, U., Fåhraeus, L., Wallentin, L. and Zador, G. (1981). Lipoprotein changes may be minimized by proper composition of a combined oral contraceptive. *Fertil. Steril.*, **35**, 172
10. Briggs, M. and Briggs, M. (1980). A randomized study of metabolic effects of four oral contraceptive preparations containing levonorgestrel plus ethinylestradiol in different regimens. In Greenblatt, R. B. (ed.) *The Development of a New Triphasic Oral Contraceptive.* pp. 79–98. (Lancaster: MTP Press)

Chapter 6

Effects of switching from higher-dose oral contraceptives to a triphasic preparation (Triquilar[R])

Th. Neufeld

INTRODUCTION

The experience gained from 20 years use of oral hormonal contraceptives has led to the development of a triphasic preparation which, while still providing excellent cycle stability, combines the advantages of administering the lowest dose of hormones just required to ensure contraception with a form of administration which is adapted to the natural cycle of the woman.

Since there is no apparent reason why the advantages of this triphasic preparation should not also be enjoyed by those women who have taken higher dosed conventional preparations – frequently for many years – we conducted a study under the conditions of daily practice to determine what effects switching a woman from higher dosed contraceptives of various composition to the triphasic preparation might have.

The main points of the study were:

(1) The cycle behavior, particularly in respect of the occurrence of intermenstrual bleeding,
(2) The general tolerance,
(3) The behavior of the body weight and blood pressure,
(4) The effect on liver function parameters,
(5) The effect on parameters of carbohydrate metabolism and, in particular, lipometabolism.

METHODS

20 women aged from 19 to 51 years with an average age of 28.3 years were recruited to the study. Heavy smokers (more than ten cigarettes per day) and greatly overweight women were excluded.

Six women had taken a higher dosed preparation for up to 3 ½ years, 14 for more than 3 ½ years. The shortest period of use was 1 ½ years, the longest 17 years.

The women were questioned in the last cycle under the old preparation and monthly under Triquilar[R], while laboratory studies were conducted in the last cycle before the switch and after 6 months use of the triphasic preparation. The switch was made on the first day of the last withdrawal bleeding.

RESULTS

Tolerance of the triphasic preparation was distinctly better than that of the previous preparations: side-effects associated with the pill, such as nausea, breast tension and vaginal discharge, were less frequent. Blemished skin improved strikingly after the switch.

The duration and intensity of withdrawal bleeding remained unchanged in 11 women, while seven reported a slight decrease of flow and two a slight increase. Withdrawal bleeding occurred after every single Triquilar[R] cycle. The fact that the reduction of the steroid dosage was not gained at the expense of an increased incidence of breakthrough bleeding or spotting merits particular mention. In a total of 120 Triquilar cycles, there was only one case of spotting and one of breakthrough bleeding – both of them in the third cycle.

The body weight (Table 1) and blood pressure values (Table 2) displayed no significant changes. The liver function para-

Table 1 Body weight values

	Pretreatment	*6th treatment cycle*	*Difference*
$\bar{x}$	55.7 kg	55.4 kg	− 0.3
t	No change		0.31 ns

Table 2 Blood pressure values

	Pretreatment	*6th treatment cycle*	*Difference*
Systolic			
$\bar{x}$	113.9 mmHg	114.5 mmHg	+ 0.6
t	No change		0.24 ns
Diastolic			
$\bar{x}$	69.5 mmHg	70.5 mmHg	+ 1.0
t	No change		0.53 ns

Table 3 Liver function parameters

	Pretreatment U/l	*6th treatment cycle U/l*	*Difference*
SGOT			
$\bar{x}$	9.4	8.5	− 0.9
t	No change		1.65 ns
SGPT			
$\bar{x}$	9.9	9.5	− 0.4
t	No change		0.48 ns

Table 4 Fasting glucose values

	Pretreatment	*6th treatment cycle*	*Difference*
$\bar{x}$	90.3 mg%	91.1 mg%	+ 0.8
t	No change		0.17 ns

Table 5 Change in lipometabolism parameters

	Pretreatment	*6th treatment cycle*	*Difference*
Total lipids			
$\bar{x}$	744.9 mg%	751.6 mg%	+ 6.7
t	Slight increase		0.22 ns
Triglycerides			
$\bar{x}$	104.6 mg%	103.8 mg%	− 0.8
t	Practically unchanged		0.10 ns
Cholesterol			
$\bar{x}$	208.0 mg%	206.5 mg%	− 1.5
t	Practically unchanged		0.27 ns

Table 6 Change in HDL-cholesterol

	Pretreatment	*6th treatment cycle*	*Difference*
HDL			
$\bar{x}$	59.4 mg%	62.7 mg%	+ 3.4
t	Slight increase		1.61 ns
$\frac{HDL}{CHOL} \times 100$			
$\bar{x}$	28.8	30.8	+ 2.0
t	Significant increase		1.84 $p < 0.1$

meters also remained unchanged. Table 3 shows the behavior of SGOT and SGPT. The fasting glucose values likewise remained unchanged (Table 4). Of particular interest is the effect of the switch on the parameters of lipometabolism (Table 5). Total lipids increase slightly, while the triglycerides and total cholesterol remain virtually unchanged. HDL-cholesterol (Table 6) shows a slight increase. We were particularly pleased to see that the HDL-cholesterol/total cholesterol quotient even increased significantly after the switch. According to general opinion, a low quotient is probably the most important risk factor for the development of arteriosclerotic cardiovascular diseases; an increase of this value must therefore be viewed as highly positive.

To summarize then, the switch does not pose any problems at all. On the contrary, cycle stability and tolerance improve, and highly positive changes occur in lipometabolism.

Chapter 7

Clinical experience with triphasic oral contraceptives (Trigynon[R]) in six hundred cycles

U. J. Gaspard, J. L. Deville and M. H. Dubois

SUMMARY

Epidemiological studies and laboratory findings now clearly indicate that adverse effects of the oral contraceptives are closely dependent on the nature and dosage of their estrogen and progestin components. In that prospect we have studied a new triphasic oral contraceptive, Trigynon[R] – Schering which contains the lowest quantity of steroids of all available preparations.

600 cycles of treatment were evaluated in 75 healthy young women (mean age: 20.7 years), of whom 70% experienced regular, normal cycles.

65% had no prior contraception while 35% were previously on combined oral contraceptives, progestin-only pills or had an IUD. The mean length of treatment with triphasic oral contraceptive was eight cycles. No pregnancy was recorded during the 600 cycles of treatment. 15% of the women dropped out of the study for medical reasons: breast tenderness, spotting, weight increase, nauseas, headaches, and leg cramps, in decreasing order of frequency. Mastalgia was present in 20% of the women under Trigynon (9.8% of the cycles), but this symptom disappeared in more than half of the cases within 3 months of oral contraceptive use.

Other side-effects were less frequent: nauseas (3.8% of the

cycles), vaginal discharge (3.8%), abdominal and leg cramps (2.8%), weight increase (3%) and headaches (2.3%).

Spotting and breakthrough bleeding accounted for only 1.8% of the cycles, a remarkably low frequency. No absence of withdrawal bleeding under Trigynon was noted in our study. Weight and blood pressure changes were minimal and never reached statistical significance.

The substantial decrease in progestin content of triphasic oral contraceptive, when compared with combined pills containing a low fixed daily dose of levonorgestrel (e.g. Microgynon[R] 30) explains why some women complain of estrogen-related symptoms such as breast tenderness and digestive disorders. However, no increase in dysmenorrhea and/or premenstrual tension was ever noted in our study. It can be concluded from this clinical evaluation that, under Trigynon, contraceptive effectiveness and control of the cycle are excellent and side-effects minimal.

This will undoubtedly increase the acceptability of low dose combined oral contraceptives.

INTRODUCTION

The latest epidemiological reports on oral contraception and its relation to diseases of the vascular system are encouraging. The Walnut Creek contraceptive drug study[1] shows no significant risk of vascular disease associated with the use of oral contraceptives. However, non-significant increases in risks of venous and arterial disease appear to be accounted for by a synergistic effect between current oral contraceptive use and heavy smoking. By contrast, the Royal College of General Practitioners' (RCGP) contraception study continues to show, as earlier[2], an excess mortality rate in oral contraceptives ever-users due to diseases of the circulatory system. However, this risk is not associated any more with duration of oral contraceptive use and it is considerably less in each age group for non-smokers than for smokers using the pill.

Other epidemiological studies clearly indicate that the risk of venous thromboembolism in oral contraception users is associated with the dose of estrogen[3] and that the change to pills containing less than 50 μg of ethinyl estradiol[4] has led to a substantial decline in venous problems. Moreover, observations have been made implying that progestogens may contribute to the increased risk of cardiovascular diseases associated with combined estrogen–progestogen oral contraceptives. A significant positive association between the dose and potency of progestogens and hypertension[5] and also deaths from stroke and ischemic heart disease has been established[6, 7].

In addition, laboratory findings are consistent with these epidemiological studies and clearly indicate that the doses of estrogens and progestogens contained in the pill are positively correlated with alterations of blood coagulation parameters, glucose and lipid metabolism[8], all factors potentially implicated in the pathogenesis of cardiovascular disorders.

In that prospect, contraceptives with low doses of estrogen and progestogen are highly desirable[9]. However, previous attempts to achieve this aim with low doses of levonorgestrel in combined pills have been hampered by difficulties in adequately controlling the cycle and, in some instances, ovulation. The new triphasic pills contain one of the lowest possible doses of ethinyl estradiol and levonorgestrel: by comparison with the lowest fixed daily dose pills containing the same steroids, triphasic pills contain 8% more ethinyl estradiol and 39% less levonorgestrel. The progestogen is given incrementally (50 μg for 6 days followed by 75 μg for the next 5 days and 125 μg for the last 10 days) while ethinyl estradiol doses are 30, 40 and again 30 μg respectively for the same periods of time.

These triphasic pills containing low doses of progestogen during the first days and providing a slight increase in ethinyl estradiol concentrations from the seventh to the eleventh days (in some way mimicking gonadal steroids fluctuations during the menstrual çycle), seem to be effective in achieving a much better control of the cycle altogether with excellent inhibition of ovulation, in spite of their reduced steroid content.

In this study, we report the clinical assessment of 600 cycles in 75 young women taking a triphasic oral contraceptive Trigynon. One particularity of the population under investigation is that 68% of the volunteers were less than 20 years of age (18.8 years). This is an interesting consideration, as far as the control of the cycle under oral contraceptive administration is concerned, in view of the frequent cycle irregularities encountered in teenage girls[8].

CHARACTERISTICS OF THE POPULATION STUDIED

Prior to the introduction in this study, women were selected on the basis of their meeting the requirements for the prescription of oral contraceptives in accordance with established medical practice. 75 normal healthy volunteers gave their informed consent to the study; 42 were recruited from the outpatient clinic of the OB/GYN department of our institution, while 33 came from the Psychosexual Information Service of our university and were assessed by the same investigators.

The test preparation Trigynon, was given with the following instructions: intake from the first package was to start on the first day of the cycle. After finishing the first calendar package, an interval of 7 days had to be observed before starting the next package.

Table 1 summarizes the number of treatment cycles considered in this study. The medication was used by 75 women for 600 cycles, i.e. a mean of eight cycles per woman.

Some relevant clinical features of the volunteers are given in Table 2: 68% of the population were under 20 years of age and the overall mean age of the women studied was 20.7 years. 72%

of the volunteers displayed a regular cycle, essentially of 24–32 days length. Volume and duration of menstruation were comprised in normal limits according to Abraham[10]. The mean age of menarche of this population was 12.97 years, which is quite normal by European criteria[11]. 5% of the women had experienced menarche at 15 and 16 years of age.

Table 1 Duration of treatment with triphasic oral contraceptive

Length of treatment	*Number of women*	%
< 3 cycles	2	2.7
3–5 cycles	33	44
6–8 cycles	24	32
9–11 cycles	5	6.7
> 12 cycles	11	14.6

Table 2 Clinical features of the volunteers

	Number of women	%	*Mean age by category of age* (y)
(a) *Age* (y)			
< 20	51	68	18.8
21–25	18	24	21.9
26–30	2	2.7	26.5
> 30	4	5.3	35.2
Total	75	(100)	20.7
(b) *Reproduction history*			
Nulligravidas	67	89.3	
Paras one or more	8	10.7	
(c) *Regularity and length of the cycle prior to contraception* (n=71)			
Irregular cycle	20	28.2	
Regular cycle	51	71.8	
length (days)	1	1.4	
< 24	1	1.4	
24–27	6	8.4	
28	21	29.6	
29–32	22	31.0	
> 32	1	1.4	

The type of contraception used by these women and, where relevant, the reasons for changing from previous contraception to triphasic oral contraception are given in Tables 3 and 4.

Table 3 Contraception used prior to the study (n=75)

	Number of women	%
No contraception	49	65.5
Progestogen only: high dose	1	1.3
low dose	3	4
IUD	2	2.7
Combined oral contraceptives	20	27

Table 4 Reasons for changing to triphasics

Previous contraception	*Reason*	*Number of women*
Progestogen-only high dose	medical reason	1
low dose	spotting	1
	no withdrawal bleeding	1
	ovarian cyst	1
IUD	spotting	1
	expulsion	1
Combined oral contraceptives	spotting	11
	no withdrawal bleeding	2
	breast tenderness	6
	nauseas, vomiting	4
	headaches	4
	excess weight gain	3
	dysmenorrhea	1

The rather young mean age of the population under investigation explains the frequent absence of prior contraception. In women changing from fixed daily dose combined oral contraceptives to triphasics, failure of adequate control of the cycle is a prominent reason for changing, much more than gastrointestinal troubles or other reasons.

RESULTS

The frequency of side-effects was 52% (39 women) under triphasic oral contraceptive administration. No pregnancy was recorded during the 600 cycles of the study. Among reasons for stopping triphasic oral contraception, personal reasons appear in one case and side-effects in 11 cases, i.e. in 16% of the population studied. The side-effects were carefully recorded during triphasic oral contraceptive administration and are summarized in Table 5. Their frequency is expressed by women and by cycles.

Table 5 Summary of side-effects under triphasic oral contraception by women and by cycles

	Number of women	*%*	*Number of cycles*	*%*
Breast tension	15	20	59	9.8
Nauseas, vomiting	6	8	23	3.8
Vaginal discharge	8	10.7	23	3.8
Abdominal and leg cramps	5	6.7	17	2.8
Excess weight	4	5.3	18	3
Headaches	4	5.3	14	2.3
Spotting + breakthrough bleeding	5	6.7	11	1.8
Dysmenorrhea	2	2.7	9	1.5
Acne	2	2.7	6	1
Depression	1	1.3	4	0.7
Appetite increase	1	1.3	3	0.5

Breast tenderness was the most frequent side-effect recorded, in almost 10% of the total number of treatment cycles, and it affected 20% of the women under study. The tendency of this symptom to improve was observed in more than half of the cases within 3 months use of triphasic oral contraception (see below). Other signs of estrogenic dominance, such as gastrointestinal disturbances, vaginal discharge, pelvic congestion and leg cramps, are also present, but much less prominent than breast tenderness. Some signs of premenstrual tension, usually ascribed to estrogen excess, such as edema, bloating, emotional instability, irritability, nervousness, depression and decreased libido, are very rare or absent.

Spotting and breakthrough bleeding show a remarkably low frequency, the latter accounting for less than 10% of intermenstrual bleeding under triphasic oral contraception. It is also noteworthy that normal withdrawal bleeding occurred after each cycle of triphasic oral contraceptive administration.

The major side-effects under triphasic oral contraceptives reported above were analyzed according to their time of onset and duration.

It was observed that most of the symptoms appeared in the first 3 months and either led to discontinuation of oral contraceptive use or, more usually, to rapid improvement or disappearance of the symptoms and continuation of use. 15 patients (20%) presented with mastalgia for 59 cycles (9.8%). The onset of this symptom appeared during the first month of triphasic contraception in nine patients, but by 3 months of treatment breast tenderness also disappeared in nine of the 15 patients. Mastalgia occurred mainly during the second (seven patients) and third phase (six patients) of oral contraceptive administration during the cycle. Figure 1a shows the decreasing frequency of this symptom with time of triphasic oral contraceptive use.

Of the 15 women with mastalgia, six dropped out within 9 months of triphasic contraception, six others experienced spontaneous improvement and disappearance of the breast symptoms and went on with the study, while the three remaining patients were lost to follow-up.

Nauseas and vomiting were experienced by six patients (8%) for 23 cycles (3.8%). In five of the six patients the onset of the symptoms occurred in the first month of treatment and improved rapidly thereafter (Figure 1b). Only one patient dropped out of the study for that reason.

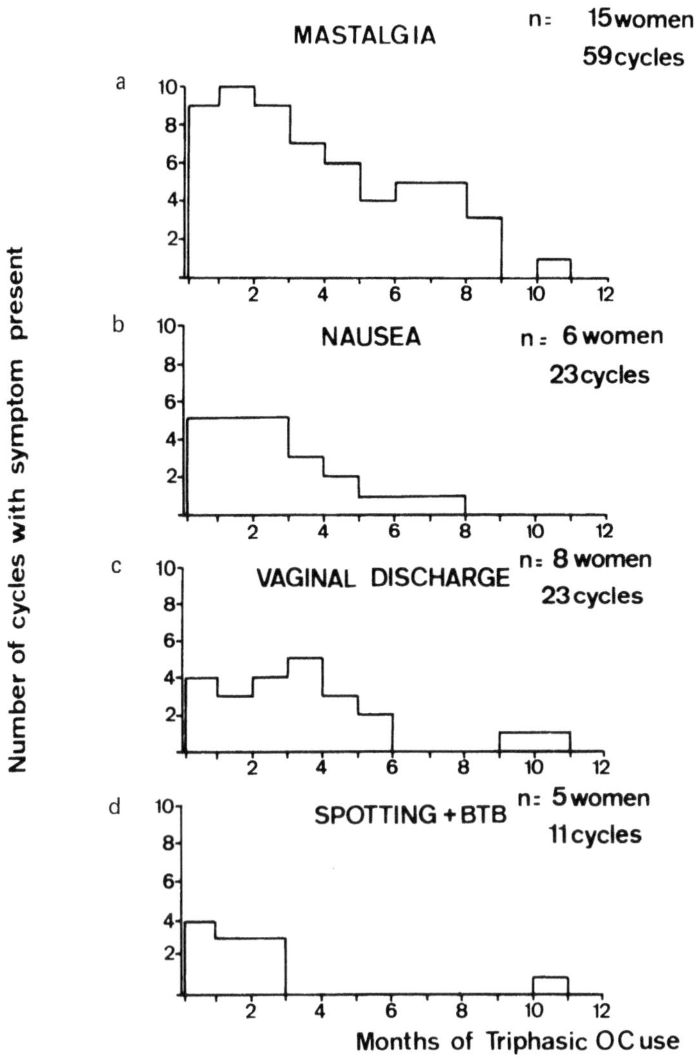

Figure 1 Number of cycles with mastalgia (a), nausea (b), vaginal discharge (c) and spotting + breakthrough bleeding (d) in relation to the duration of triphasic oral contraceptive use

Vaginal discharge was present in eight patients (10.6%) for 23 cycles (3.8%). In five of the eight patients the onset of this symptom occurred in the first months of treatment. Figure 1c shows the frequency of this symptom with time of oral contraceptive use. No patient dropped out of the study for that reason. Spotting and breakthrough bleeding (BTB) occurred only in five patients (6.6%) for 11 cycles (1.8%). In four patients spotting or BTB appeared initially in the first months of treatment and quickly improved thereafter as can be seen in Figure 1d. Two patients dropped out of the study for BTB.

Table 6 Changes in weight and arterial blood pressure during triphasic oral contraception

	Before treatment	*During triphasic oral contraceptive administration*		
		3rd month	*6th month*	*12th month*
Number of women	75	56	38	11
Weight (kg)	55.8 ± 0.9* (45–71.5)	56.6 ± 1.1 (46–69)	55.3 ± 1.2 (47–69)	57.7 ± 2.1 (48–68)
Systolic BP(mmHg)	121 ± 3 (100–145)	122 ± 1 (100–140)	122 ± 3 (100–145)	123 ± 4 (100–140)
Diastolic BP(mmHg)	76 ± 1 (60–95)	77 ± 1 (60–90)	75 ± 2 (60–90)	81 ± 3 (60–90)

*Mean ± SEM, and ( ) range. All differences between groups and individuals are not statistically significant (Student's *t*-test for non-paired and paired values)

Changes in weight, systolic and diastolic arterial blood pressure, are given in Table 6. Absence of change in weight was recorded in one third of the women while another third experienced a weight reduction from 1 to 4 kg and the last third gained from 1 to 4 kg. Three women dropped out of the study for a weight gain that they subjectively rated as excessive. Statistical analyses of weight fluctuations at different intervals of time during treatment showed no significant difference between groups or individuals, according to Student's *t*-test for non-paired and paired values, respectively.

Lack of statistically significant variations in either systolic or diastolic blood pressure values was also observed.

Blood pressure values remained practically constant and in no case was it necessary to discontinue medication prematurely for that reason.

Table 7 Comparison of side-effects before* and during triphasic oral contraception

	Before triphasic oral contraception		*During triphasic oral contraception*	
	Number of women	%	*Number of women*	%
Breast tension	6	8	15	20†
Nauseas, vomiting	4	5.3	6	8
Vaginal discharge	1	1.3	8	10.7†
Abdominal and leg cramps	0	0	5	6.7†
Excess weight	3	4	4	5.3
Headaches	4	5.3	4	5.3
Spotting + BTB	14	18.7†	5	6.7
Dysmenorrhea	3	4	2	2.7
Acne	0	0	2	2.7
Appetite increase	0	0	1	1.3
Depression	0	0	1	1.3
No withdrawal bleeding	1	1.3	0	0

*including 24 women on previous oral contraception (=32%)
† $p < 0.05$ by chi square analysis

Different symptoms carefully recorded in our group of volunteers before initiation of the study and during triphasic oral contraceptive administration were compared (Table 7). It must be remembered that 32% of the women were on oral contraception before changing to triphasic pill. Chi square analysis shows that a significant increase in the frequency of breast tension, vaginal discharge and abdominal and leg cramps is observed under triphasic treatment ($p < 0.05$). By contrast, spotting and breakthrough bleeding are distinctly and significantly improved when switching to triphasic oral contraception.

Table 8 summarizes the side-effects which led 11 of the women studied to discontinue triphasic oral contraception: breast discomfort is by far the main reason for dropping out.

Table 8 Side-effects leading to discontinuation of triphasic oral contraception

	Number of women	*%*
Breast tension	6	8
Spotting	2	2.7
Excess weight	3	4
Nauseas, vomiting	1	1.3
Headaches	1	1.3
Leg cramps	1	1.3
Depression	1	1.3

Table 9 shows that the continuation rate under triphasic oral contraception is significantly decreased in women who already had discontinued previous combined fixed daily dose oral contraceptives.

Table 9 Continuation rate under triphasic oral contraception vs previous contraception

Previous contraception	*Continuation on triphasic*		*Discontinuation*	
	Number of women	*%*	*Number of women*	*%*
No contraception	45	92	4	8
IUD or progestogen only	5	83	1	17
Combined oral contraceptives (fixed dose)	13	65*	7	35

*$\chi^2 = 22.1$, $p < 0.0001$

DISCUSSION

A general consensus is now reached that the oral contraceptive of choice for the majority of women has to contain the lowest dose of estrogen and progestogen compatible with maximum contraceptive effectiveness, optimum safety and patient acceptability[9,12].

The triphasic combination Trigynon contains the lowest total quantity of steroids of all available preparations and it is therefore of great interest to determine whether this type of triphasic combination compares advantageously or not with low fixed dose combinations which are hampered by suboptimal control of the cycle[13,14]. 100% protection against conception has been observed in our study of 600 cycles under triphasic medication and this result is in complete agreement with the report of Lachnit-Fixson that no pregnancy occurred in 8068 treatment cycles under the same oral contraceptive[14] despite medication errors and one or several omissions of tablets.

Trigynon inhibits ovulation and reduces the cervical score in a very effective way[15]. However, some pregnancies apparently related to drug failure have recently been reported[16]. Accordingly, it must be stressed that owing to the reduction of steroid dosage and to the triphasic nature of this combination, women should be careful to avoid tablet omission and to take the preparation stepwise.

The control of the cycle achieved in our study is quite remarkable. The addition of the number of cycles where breakthrough bleeding and spotting occurred (expressed as percentages of the total number of treatment cycles) is 1.8%. These results are distinctly better than those reported by Lachnit-Fixson[14] and Zador[13] which amount to 8–10% of the cycles.

It is noteworthy that in the study of Zador[13], comparison of triphasic oral contraception with a low fixed dose combined oral contraceptive (Microgynon[R] 30, ethinyl estradiol 30 μg + levonorgestrel 150 μg) points to suboptimal control of the cycle with the latter preparation: 15.7% of the cycles were presenting with spotting and/or breakthrough bleeding.

We also report a clearcut and statistically significant improvement in the control of the cycle (Table 7) when women change from no previous contraception, or from other types of contraception, to triphasic oral contraceptives.

Withdrawal bleeding is always observed after each cycle of triphasic oral contraceptive administration and the results obtained are much better than with low fixed dose oral contraceptives[13,14].

In keeping with other observations[9] our results support the view that triphasic preparations are relatively estrogen-dominant. Indeed, 20% of the women in our study complain of breast tenderness (9.8% of total number of treatment cycles), a frequency almost twice as high as the one reported previously[13,14] and 3.7 times greater than the one observed[13] under Microgynon 30. As indicated by Lachnit-Fixson[17] breast discomfort improves rather impressively with time and this is confirmed by our study. Discontinuation of triphasic oral contraception is more often related to this symptom than to any other (see Table 8). Other signs usually more or less related to estrogen dominance, such as gastrointestinal disturbances, abdominal and leg cramps, and vaginal discharge, are encountered with a rather low frequency. However, irritability, nervousness, bloating, tension headaches, which all are symptoms frequently related to the premenstrual tension syndrome and more likely to occur under an estrogen-dominant preparation[18], are either absent or uncommon in the population we studied.

Weight changes and blood pressure fluctuations are very slight under triphasic oral contraception and not statistically significant. In three instances, however, a weight increase of less than 4 kg caused the patients to drop out of the study. It is noteworthy that a rather equivalent number of women either gained or lost weight during the study.

CONCLUSION

From our clinical assessment of 600 cycles under triphasic oral contraception in 75 young women, and in agreement with other clinical studies, it can be clearly stated that the triphasic preparation Trigynon offers a very reliable protection against conception and that its tolerance and cycle control are optimal in spite of the very low content of steroids in this preparation. Particularly, the very low frequency of spotting, breakthrough bleeding and amenorrhea obtained under triphasic pills constitutes substantial improvement over combined pills containing a low fixed dose of steroids. This improvement is liable to increase the acceptability of low dose oral contraception. The substantial decrease in progestogen content in triphasic pills explains why some patients complain of estrogen-related symptoms (breast tenderness, digestive disorders, vaginal discharge, abdominal and leg cramps). In our study, these symptoms usually improved rapidly and they only led to discontinuation of triphasic oral contraception in about 10% of the women. Altogether, with reports indicating minimal impact of triphasic pills on coagulation parameters, glucose tolerance and lipid profile (especially HDL-cholesterol concentration[19]), the excellent results concerning the contraceptive effectiveness and control of the cycle allow us to consider this new type of triphasic low dose contraception as interesting. This may be especially true in subgroups of women with increased risk under oral contraception such as teenagers and women over 35 years of age, particularly women who smoke. However, owing to the slight estrogen dominance of this preparation it should not be administered to women presenting with benign breast disease[9].

ACKNOWLEDGEMENTS

The authors thank Mrs A. M. Verly-Smolnik for her collaboration in the preparation of the manuscript.

References

1. Ramcharan, S., Pellegrin, F. A., Ray, R. M. and Hsu, J. (1980). The Walnut Creek contraceptive drug study. A prospective study of the side effects of oral contraceptives. *J. Reprod. Med.*, **25**, 346
2. Royal College of General Practitioners' Oral contraception study (1981). Further analyses of mortality in oral contraceptive users. *Lancet*, **2**, 542
3. Inman, W. H. W., Vessey, M. P., Westerholm, B. and Engerlund, A. (1970). Thromboembolic disease and the steroidal content of oral contraceptives. A report to the Committee on Safety of drugs. *Br. Med. J.*, **11**, 20
4. Bottiger, I. E., Boman, G., Eklund, G. and Westerholm, B. (1980). Oral contraceptives and thromboembolic disease: effects of lowering oestrogen content. *Lancet*, **1**, 1096
5. Royal College of General Practitioners' Oral contraception study (1977). Effect on hypertension and benign breast disease of progestogen component in combined oral contraceptives. *Lancet*, **1**, 624
6. Kay, C. R. (1980). The happiness pill? *J. R. Coll. Gen. Pract.*, **30**, 8
7. Meade, T. W., Greenberg, G. and Thompson, S. G. (1980). Progestogens and cardiovascular reactions associated with oral contraceptives and a comparison of the safety of 50 and 30 μg oestrogen preparations. *Br. Med. J.*, **280**, 1157
8. Briggs, M. H. and Briggs, M. (1980). A randomized study of metabolic effects of four oral contraceptive preparations containing levonorgestrel plus ethinyloestradiol in different regimens. In Greenblatt, R. B. (ed.) *The Development of a New Triphasic Oral Contraceptive*. pp. 79–98. (Lancaster: MTP Press)
9. Editorial (1981). Triphasic oral contraceptives. *Lancet*, **1**, 1191
10. Abraham, G. E. (1978). The normal menstrual cycle. In Givens, J. R. (ed.) *Endocrine Causes of Menstrual Disorders*. pp. 15–44. (Chicago: Year Book Medical Publishers)
11. Dewhurst, C. J. (1980). *Practical Paediatric and Adolescent Gynecology*. p. 272. (New York: Marcel Dekker)
12. Spellacy, W. N., Buhi, W. C. and Birk, S. A. (1981). Prospective studies of carbohydrate metabolism in 'normal' women using norgestrel for eighteen months. *Fertil. Steril.*, **35**, 167
13. Zador, G. (1979). Fertility regulation using 'triphasic' administration of ethinylestradiol and levonorgestrel in comparison with the 30 plus 150 μg fixed dose regime. *Acta Obstet. Gynecol. Scand.*, **88**, (Suppl.), 43
14. Lachnit-Fixson, U. (1979). Erstes Dreistufenpräparat zur hormonalen Konzeptionsverhütung. *Münch. Med. Wochenschr.*, **121**, 1421
15. Spona, J., Schneider, W. H. F. and Lachnit-Fixson, U. (1980). Mode of action of triphasic oral contraception. In Greenblatt, R. B. (ed.) *The Development of a New Triphasic Oral Contraceptive*. pp. 51–68. (Lancaster: MTP Press)
16. Fay, R. A. (1982). Failure with the new triphasic oral contraceptive Logynon^R. *Br. Med. J.*, **284**, 17

17. Lachnit-Fixson, U. (1980). Clinical investigation with a new triphasic oral contraceptive. In Greenblatt, R. B. (ed.) *The Development of a New Triphasic Oral Contraceptive*. pp. 99–107. (Lancaster: MTP Press)
18. Cullberg, J. (1972). Mood changes and menstrual symptoms with different gestogen/estrogen combinations. *Acta Psychiatr. Scand.*, **236** (Suppl.), 1
19. Larsson-Cohn, U., Fåhreus, L., Wallentin, L. and Zador, G. (1981). Lipoprotein changes may be minimized by proper composition of a combined oral contraceptive. *Fertil. Steril.*, **35**, 172

Chapter 8

Acceptability of low-dose oral contraceptives: results of a randomized Swedish multicenter study comparing a triphasic (Trionetta[R])* and a fixed-dose combination (Neovletta[R])**

L. Carlborg

INTRODUCTION

The contraceptive effectiveness of combined oral contraceptives has never been a great problem and failures can mainly be attributed to errors in tablet intake. For several reasons research has been directed to the reduction of hormonal content. Subjective side-effects reported by the users first promoted efforts to reduce the ingested doses. These side-effects generally subsided after discontinuation of medication and were mainly classified as trivial. A great deal of attention has been drawn to some serious, but fortunately rare side-effects. These include above all thromboembolic diseases. From the beginning the estrogen component was considered to be responsible for most of the adverse effects and appropriate reduction was made in many steps until the lowest dose was reached that was able to cause ovulation inhibition and give a good cycle control. Recent research has drawn attention to the fact that the progestogen also could be of importance with regard to serious side-effects with oral contraceptives. An increasing incidence of hypertension with increasing dose of progestogen has been reported[1]. Furthermore, progestogens belonging to the 19-nor-testosterone type are reported to have a dose-related negative effect on HDL[2, 3, 4]. It therefore seems to be highly desirable to reduce the progestogen dose in oral contraceptives.

*Also known as Triquilar[R], Trigynon[R] and Logynon[R]
**Also known as Microgynon[R] 30

A further reason for striving to reduce both estrogen and progestogen is the fact that the suppression of the hypothalamic-pituitary axis is reported to be dose dependent[5]. The risk of getting 'post pill amenorrhea' is more likely to occur when unnecessarily high doses have been administered.

When the doses in oral contraceptives are reduced the subjective side-effects reported by the users are generally diminished. Another problem is instead now paramount. Bleeding irregularities, especially in the first cycles may be of such a degree that some women abandon the pills. An unwanted pregnancy and a demand for therapeutic abortion may follow. Some low-dose oral contraceptives fail too often to give a withdrawal bleeding in the table-free week. This is of great concern for the patient and will cause unnecessary pregnancy tests.

A good way to decrease the doses is to vary the hormonal content in three phases thus mimicking the endogenous hormonal levels. At least theoretically this method would reduce bleeding irregularities as it better conforms to endometrial dynamics. The present study was undertaken to compare a new triphasic oral contraceptive with the presently most widely used monophasic preparation. The two preparations contain the same synthetic hormones, but the new formula has a considerably reduced progestogen dose. The comparison included evaluation of the overall acceptability in terms of cycle control and side-effects.

MATERIAL AND METHODS

The fixed dose preparation Neovletta[R] contains 30 μg of ethinyl estradiol and 150 μg of levonorgestrel per tablet. Trionetta[R] also consists of 21 active tablets per cycle but is subdivided in three phases: 6 tablets with 30 μg ethinyl estradiol + 50 μg levonorgestrel, followed by 5 tablets with 40 μg ethinyl estradiol + 75 μg levonorgestrel and finally 10 tablets with 30 μg ethinyl estradiol + 125 μg levonorgestrel. The total intake of levonorgestrel per cycle is decreased by 40% in Trionetta compared to Neovletta, while the estrogen dose is approximately the same. Two versions of Trionetta were studied: Trionetta 21, containing the 21 active tablets, and Trionetta 28 which in addition contains seven placebo tablets, to be taken in the corresponding tablet-free week when using the 21-tablet version. The 28-tablet version is thought to make it easier for some women to take their contraceptive pills. A total of 862 women from 12 different family planning centres in Sweden were included in the study. Generally, patients were selected on the basis of their meeting the requirements for the prescription of oral contraceptives in accordance with established medical practice. Before entering the study the women gave their verbal consent.

Out of the total number (862) 27 women (3.1%) did not come back to any follow-up visit and did not give any information to the prescriber. These patients are left out in the evaluation.

Protocols suitable for computer analysis were used. The women gave information on menstrual bleeding pattern, parity, abortions and previous contraceptive methods, before entering the study. Physical examination, including measurement of blood pressure and body weight, was also made.

The participants were allocated to the three treatment groups in a randomized fashion. 50% of the women were allocated to use Neovletta, 25% to use Trionetta 21 and 25% to use Trionetta 28. Both verbal and written instructions were given to the volunteers. They were all told to take the first tablet on the first day of the menstrual cycle.

The total patient material with respect to age distribution is shown in Table 1. As can be seen, more than 60% of the women were between 16 and 25 years in all treatment groups.

There were no differences in the patient material between the treatment groups with regard to number of previous pregnancies (Table 2) or use of hormonal contraceptives 3 months before start of trial (Table 3).

Table 1 Age distribution

Year	*Neovletta*[R]		*Trionetta*[R]		*Trionetta 21*[R]		*Trionetta 28*[R]	
	No.	*%*	*No.*	*%*	*No.*	*%*	*No.*	*%*
≤ 15	28	6.7	22	5.3	10	4.8	12	5.8
16–20	171	40.9	155	37.2	79	37.6	76	36.7
21–25	93	22.2	108	25.9	53	25.2	55	26.6
26–30	72	17.2	74	17.7	39	18.6	35	16.9
31–35	35	8.4	40	9.6	21	10.0	19	9.2
36–40	16	3.8	18	4.3	8	3.8	10	4.8
41–45	2	0.5						
46–50	1	0.2						
Total	418		417		210		207	

Table 2 Previous pregnancies (births and abortions)

	Neovletta[R]		*Trionetta*[R]		*Trionetta* [R]*21*		*Trionetta* [R]*28*	
	No.	*%*	*No.*	*%*	*No.*	*%*	*No.*	*%*
0	247	59.2	247	59.2	123	58.6	124	59.9
1	56	13.4	47	11.3	23	11.0	24	11.6
2	64	15.3	76	18.2	45	21.4	31	15.0
3	32	7.7	35	8.4	16	7.6	19	9.2
4	9	2.2	9	2.2	3	1.4	6	2.9
5	6	1.4	3	0.7			3	1.4
6	3	0.7						

Table 3 Use of hormonal contraceptives 3 months before start of trial

	Neovletta[R] (*% of women*)	*Trionetta*[R] (*% of women*)	*Trionetta* [R]*21* (*% of women*)	*Trionetta* [R]*28* (*% of women*)
Combined preparations	31.8	31.7	31.9	31.4
'Mini-pills'	1.9	2.4	1.9	2.9

Follow-up visits were requested after three, six and for some women also after 12 cycles. They reported pertinent clinical events and their body weight and blood pressure were also recorded.

Subjective complaints were recorded if reported spontaneously. Details concerning menstrual flow, breakthrough bleeding, spotting and missed tablets were recorded by the women on a special chart. Intermenstrual bleeding was classified as 'breakthrough bleeding' when the quantity of blood loss required the use of any sanitary protection, and as 'spotting' in all other cases.

'Missed withdrawal bleeding' is defined as absence of bleeding in the tablet-free interval (or when taking the placebo tablets).

Table 4 **Number of women completing each cycle**

Cycle	*Neovletta*[R]		*Trionetta*[R]		*Trionetta* [R]*21*		*Trionetta* [R]*28*	
	No.	*%*	*No.*	*%*	*No.*	*%*	*No.*	*%*
1	406	97.1	405	97.1	204	97.1	201	97.1
2	396	94.7	393	94.2	197	93.8	196	94.7
3	385	92.1	382	91.6	189	90.0	193	93.2
4	365	87.3	358	85.9	174	82.9	184	88.9
5	361	86.4	354	84.9	172	81.9	182	87.9
6	358	85.6	350	83.9	170	81.0	180	87.0
7	170	40.7	163	39.1	81	38.6	82	39.6
8	170	40.7	161	38.6	79	37.6	82	39.6
9	168	40.2	160	38.4	78	37.1	82	39.6
10	166	39.7	158	37.9	77	36.7	81	39.1
11	165	39.5	157	37.6	77	36.7	80	38.6
12	165	39.5	156	37.4	76	36.2	80	38.6
Total number of cycles	3275		3197		1574		1623	

RESULTS

The 835 women completed a total number of 6472 cycles. The distribution of the patients in relation to the number of cycles completed is shown in Table 4. As can be seen the number of women completing each cycle was almost the same for both formulations, being approximately 85% in the first trial period of 6 months. The figure for Trionetta 28 (87.9%) is slightly higher than for Trionetta 21 (81.9%). In the group of 371 women being scheduled for additional six cycles the distribution was similar for the test preparations.

Efficacy

In this study there was a comparatively high number of missed tablets. Tablets were omitted in 8.1% of the total number of cycles in the triphasic group and the corresponding figure for the monophasic group was 9.4%.

In spite of this fact only one pregnancy occurred during the observation period and during treatment with Trionetta 21. This pregnancy was classified by the attending physician as clearly due to patient failure (3 consecutively missed tablets).

Cycle control

Cycle length

Both formulations exerted a normalizing effect on cycle length, this effect being more pronounced with the triphasic formulation. The last untreated cycle was reported as being 28 ± 2 days for 81.4% of the women in the Neovletta group and 76.9% in the Trionetta group. In the 6th and 12th treatment cycle the corresponding figures were 89.2% and 90.4% respectively for Neovletta and for Trionetta 94.5% and 94.2% respectively. The cycle regulating effect was particularly seen in women who previously had shorter, longer or completely irregular cycle intervals.

Duration of bleeding

The two combinations reduced to the same extent previously prolonged bleeding periods (>7 days). The percentage of women with bleeding periods longer than 7 days in the 6th and 12th treatment cycle was 1.4% and 0.6% respectively for Neovletta and 0.9% and 0.6% respectively for Trionetta. The percentage of women with very short bleeding periods (<4 days) was unchanged in the Trionetta group while there was an increase from 7.7% (last untreated cycle) to 17.9% in the 12th cycle in the Neovletta group. Thus the proportion of women with a 'normal' duration of bleeding (4–7 day-interval) increased during treatment with Trionetta.

Intensity of bleeding

The amount of menstrual flow was defined by the participants as 'scanty', 'normal' or 'profuse'. The menstrual flow was reduced during the treatment. The two combinations reduced to the same extent previously profuse bleedings. In the last untreated cycle the percentage of women with profuse bleeding was 6.7% in the Neovletta group and 9.1% in the Trionetta group. In the 6th and 12th treatment cycle the corresponding figures were 0.9% and 1.2% respectively for Neovletta and 0.6% and 1.3% respectively for Trionetta. However, 'scanty' bleeding was reported more frequently by women using Neovletta than by women using Trionetta. Normal bleeding was more often reported during treatment with Trionetta.

Missed withdrawal bleeding

Failure of withdrawal bleeding (missed withdrawal bleeding being defined as absence of bleeding during the tablet-free interval) to occur was rare in both treatment groups but the triphasic formulation was found to be superior to the fixed dose combination. Calculated in relation to the total number of cycles, withdrawal bleeding did not occur in 20 cycles out of 3197 cycles (=0.6%) in women taking Trionetta and in 74 cycles out of 3275 cycles (=2.3%) in women taking Neovletta. This difference is statistically significant ($p<0.05$, Fisher's test).

Intermenstrual bleeding

The pattern of intermenstrual bleeding – spotting/breakthrough bleeding in percentage of cycles – in the last untreated cycle and during treatment is shown in Table 5.

Table 5 Intermenstrual bleeding before and during treatment

	Neovletta[R] (*% of cycles*)	*Trionetta*[R] (*% of cycles*)	*Trionetta* [R]*21* (*% of cycles*)	*Trionetta* [R]*28* (*% of cycles*)
Last untreated cycle				
Spotting	4.8	5.0	5.7	4.4
Breakthrough bleeding	1.4	1.7	2.4	1.0
1st to 3rd cycle				
Spotting	15.8	9.0	10.5	7.5
Breakthrough bleeding	6.3	3.1	3.9	2.4
4th to 6th cycle				
Spotting	7.4	5.0	6.0	4.0
Breakthrough bleeding	4.8	3.6	5.2	2.0
7th to 12th cycle				
Spotting	5.0	3.4	3.8	2.5
Breakthrough bleeding	2.2	1.2	1.3	1.0
1st to 12th cycle				
Spotting	9.7	6.0	7.2	4.8
Breakthrough bleeding	4.5	2.7	3.6	1.9

Prior to treatment the frequency of intermenstrual bleeding was almost the same in both treatment groups: Neovletta 6.2% and Trionetta 6.7%. During the treatment a marked difference between the two formulations was found. In spite of the fact that the triphasic formulation contains a considerably lower dose of hormones this preparation was superior to the fixed dose combination in terms of a lower frequency of intermenstrual bleeding. Especially during the critical first months of use the difference was most obvious. The incidence of spotting and breakthrough bleeding during the first three cycles was 15.8% and 6.3% respectively for Neovletta and 9.0% and 3.1% respectively for Trionetta.

Even when calculated on the total number of cycles (1st to 12th cycle) the difference between the two formulations is evident. The incidence of spotting and breakthrough bleeding with this calculation was 9.7% and 4.5% respectively for Neovletta and 6.0% and 2.7% respectively for Trionetta. This difference is statistically significant ($p<0.05$, Fisher's test).

As can be seen from Table 5 there was a tendency for the 28-pack version (Trionetta 28) to give a lower frequency of intermenstrual bleeding compared to the 21-pack version. A possible reason for this could be a more regular tablet intake with Trionetta 28.

Table 6 Intermenstrual bleeding during treatment

	Neovletta[R] *(% of cycles)*	*Trionetta*[R] *(% of cycles)*
No tablets omitted*		
Spotting	8.6	5.3
Breakthrough bleeding	3.7	2.3
Tablets omitted**		
Spotting	19.8	13.2
Breakthrough bleeding	12.0	7.8
Total		
Spotting	9.7	6.0
Breakthrough bleeding	4.5	2.7

*Number of cycles: Neovletta 2967, Trionetta 2939
**Number of cycles: Neovletta 308, Trionetta 258

Table 6 shows how important correct intake of medication is for good cycle control. Spotting and especially breakthrough bleeding occur considerably more frequently in cycles with intake errors.

Patient withdrawal

As can be seen from Table 7 the continuation of treatment was similar in both treatment groups. In the Neovletta group 85.9%

Table 7 Continuation/withdrawal

	Neovletta^{R}		*Trionetta*^{R}		*Trionetta*^{R}*21*		*Trionetta*^{R}*28*	
	*Cycle 1–6** (*% of women*)	*Cycle 7–12*** (*% of women*)	*Cycle 1–6** (*% of women*)	*Cycle 7–12*** (*% of women*)	*Cycle 1–6** (*% of women*)	*Cycle 7–12*** (*% of women*)	*Cycle 1–6** (*% of women*)	*Cycle 7–12*** (*% of women*)
Continued	85.9	87.3	83.9	85.7	81.0	85.4	87.0	86.0
Discontinued	14.1	12.7	16.1	14.3	19.0	14.6	13.0	14.0
Medical reasons	8.6	9.0	11.3	8.8	13.8	7.9	8.7	9.7
Personal reasons	5.7	4.2	5.3	5.5	6.2	6.7	4.4	4.3

*Number of women: Neovletta 418
Trionetta 417
Trionetta 21 210
Trionetta 28 207

**Number of women: Neovletta 189
Trionetta 182
Trionetta 21 89
Trionetta 28 93

completed the first trial period of six cycles. The corresponding figure for Trionetta was 83.9%. Of the participants scheduled for an additional control after 12 cycles of treatment 87.3% in the Neovletta group completed 12 cycles of treatment. The corresponding figure for Trionetta was 85.7%.

The most common medical reasons for discontinuing treatment with Neovletta were: intermenstrual bleeding (5.3%), nausea, vomiting (1.9%), headache (1.9%) and depression (1.2%). The most common medical reasons for discontinuing treatment with Trionetta was: intermenstrual bleeding (4.1%), nausea, vomiting (2.6%), headache (2.2%) and increased withdrawal bleeding (1.7%).

One patient taking Neovletta and two patients taking Trionetta discontinued because of hypertension.

Table 8 Side-effects reported in more than 1% of the cycles

	Neovletta[R]		*Trionetta*[R]	
	Last untreated cycle (%)	*During treatment (%)*	*Last untreated cycle (%)*	*During treatment (%)*
Dysmenorrhea				
slight	24.9	11.3	27.3	16.1
severe	10.5	2.2	14.6	1.9
Acne	9.8	4.1	8.9	4.5
Headache	4.8	3.9	3.8	3.2
migrainous	1.7	0.5	1.4	1.6
Nausea, vomiting	1.2	1.2	1.4	2.3
Breast tension	2.2	1.8	0.7	1.7
Depression	0.5	0.9	1.0	1.4

Side-effects

Side-effects reported in more than 1% of the treatment cycles are shown in Table 8. Acne and headache were for both formulations reported less frequently during treatment than in the last untreated cycle. Although these data must be evaluated with due reservation, it can be said that both formulations are very well tolerated.

One case of thrombophlebitis was reported during treatment with Neovletta.

There was no statistically significant increase of the mean blood pressure or the mean body weight during treatment.

CONCLUSION

From the results of this comparative clinical trial it can be concluded that both formulations are highly effective and well tolerated oral contraceptives.

The new concept of decreasing the total content of ingested hormones in an oral contraceptive in a three-step fashion which mimics the endogenous hormone levels in a menstrual cycle has been shown to be very successful.

The good cycle control already brought about by the fixed dose combination of levonorgestrel and ethinyl estradiol (Neovletta) in comparison to other low-dose oral contraceptives[6,7] has been further improved by the three-step formulation (Trionetta) using the same compounds.

This has been achieved along with the benefit of a significantly reduced steroid content.

Trionetta is thus considered to be the first choice among oral contraceptives.

ACKNOWLEDGEMENT

The author would like to express his gratitude to the following gynecologists and midwives:

Eskilstuna: Carl-Axel Ingemanson, Ann-Cathrin Lindblad and Vivi-Ann Westman
Gällivare: Hans Frykman and Ewa Sjölander
Halmstad: Birgitta Gullbrandsson and Sven-Olov Sandström
Helsingborg: Kjell Andersson and Annika Nordlund

Karlstad:	Arne Eliasson and Märta Holmqvist
Lidköping:	Gudrun Broberg, Anita Brännström, Barbro Jenschke, Bengt Klang, Ingemar Klinte and Hans Westholm
Mjölby:	Ann-Margreth Nordgren and Rigmor Stahre
Varberg:	Isac Bachrach and Britta Johansson
Vänersborg:	Rolf Bengtsson, Sonia Bergström and Berit Svensson
Värnamo:	Adam Sydsjö and Irene Winbladh
Västervik:	Helena Andersson, Gudrun Folke, Annica Gustafsson, Magnus Jägerhorn and May-Lis Loftås
Västerås:	Marie-Ann Frelén and Göran Lidbjörk

References

1. Wingrave, S. J. (1982). Progestogen effects and their relationship to lipoprotein changes. A report from the Oral Contraception Study of the Royal College of General Practitioners. *Acta Obstet. Gynecol. Scand.*, 105 (Suppl.), 33
2. Larsson-Cohn, U., Fåhraeus, L., Wallentin, L. and Zador, G. (1981). Lipoprotein changes may be minimized by proper composition of a combined oral contraceptive. *Fertil. Steril.*, **35**, 172
3. Larsson-Cohn, U., Wallentin, L. and Zador, G. (1979). Plasma lipids and high density lipoproteins during oral contraception with different combinations of ethinyl estradiol and levonorgestrel. *Horm. Metab. Res.*, **11**, 437
4. Briggs, M. H. and Briggs, M. (1982). Randomized prospective studies on metabolic effects of oral contraceptives. *Acta Obstet. Gynecol. Scand.*, 105 (Suppl.), 25
5. Spellacy, W. N., Kalra, P. S., Buhi, W. C. and Birk, S. A. (1980). Pituitary and ovarian responsiveness to a graded gonadotropin releasing factor stimulation test in women using a low-estrogen or a regular type of oral contraceptive. *Am. J. Obstet. Gynecol.*, **137**, 109
6. Bergstein, N. A. M. (1976). Clinical efficacy, acceptability and metabolic effects of new low dose combined oral contraceptives. *Acta Obstet. Gynecol. Scand.*, 54 (Suppl.), 51
7. Borglin, N. E. (1980). Experience of Restovar^{R}, a new combined contraceptive pill of low hormonal potency. *Curr. Ther. Res.*, **27**, 88

Discussion

Question Has Dr Zador any evidence from further cycles of treatment that have occurred in the time interval since his paper was prepared?

Dr Zador Yes, there has emerged a consistency of opinion from both gynecologists and nurses and midwives (who are prescribing the pill) that the triphasic pill continues to be well accepted. Could I also point out that, although the findings of both Dr Carlborg and myself are similar, we have never actually discussed the mutual consistency of our separate findings before with regard to breakthrough bleeding.

Question What are the consequences of a patient forgetting more than one pill when on the triphasic pill in comparison to the same error when the patient is using a fixed low-dose pill?

Dr Zador It is well recognized that low-dose omission may invite ovulation, as might decreased absorbtion or accelerated metabolism. Thus forgetting one tablet in the first half of the cycle might be deleterious. However appropriate counselling of the patient is necessary. The majority of the hitherto reported cases of pregnancy have all occurred due to patient failure.

Question Could the high frequency of spotting in the first cycle, which you reported, be explained by the day of the cycle chosen for treatment to start?

Dr Zador In our study, on the first day of the triphasic comparative studies, all women were instructed to start on day five. It was a later recommendation by the manufacturers that treatment should start on day one. The starting day does not however seem to influence the frequency of bleeding irregularities.

Question Does Dr Gaspard not agree that any apparent lack of effect on blood pressure is not significant if it is only assessed after 12 months since hypertensive effects only tend to occur with longer pill usage? Is not longer experience necessary?

Dr Gaspard I agree. However, other investigators have not been able to observe any significant fluctuations of blood pressure during longer periods of treatment with triphasic oral contraceptives.

Question Would not the incidence of breast tenderness be increased by the fact that 65% of your patient studies had not, prior to study, used oral contraception?

Dr Gaspard Breast tenderness in the population we studied was positively correlated with the younger age spectrum of the volunteers. It was elevated only in those who had not used oral contraception before.

Question Does Dr Neufeld feel that a woman on a 50 μg tablet – who is not experiencing any side-effects – should be switched to a low-dose preparation?

Dr Neufeld If a preparation containing a lower dose of active compound gives the same clinical effect as that of a higher dose, then the lower dose should be used.

Question What are Dr Neufeld's medical reasons for discontinuation of the pill?

Dr Neufeld Any sign of thromboembolic disease, even superficial phlebitis or any increase in blood pressure.

Section III

Metabolism and the Hemostatic System

Moderator: K. Irsigler

Chapter 9

Lipoproteins and the estrogenicity of oral contraceptives

U. Larsson-Cohn

SUMMARY

After a very brief discussion about plasma lipids and lipoproteins the results are summarized of a recent clinical investigation concerned with effects of four different ethinyl estradiol/levonorgestrel combinations on SHBG and on some plasma lipids and lipoproteins.

There is a very good correlation between the ethinyl estradiol/levonorgestrel ratios of the drugs and their effects on the plasma levels of SHBG. The levonorgestrel-dominated drugs, i.e. the combinations 20/250 and 30/250, significantly reduce the HDL-cholesterol, the 'good cholesterol', while 30/150 and Triquilar^{R} have only small effects in that respect.

It is concluded that it seems to be the total estrogenicity of an ethinyl estradiol/levonorgestrel combination that determines the effects on plasma lipoproteins and that, by carefully balancing the two components against each other, it is possible to minimize the consequences of such a combination on plasma lipids and lipoproteins.

INTRODUCTION

The rate of cardiovascular disease is influenced by many factors such as age, gender, blood pressure, physical activity, nutrition, smoking habits, alcohol intake etc. and also by the concentrations in plasma of cholesterol and triglycerides. Most investigators in this field have found that high levels of cholesterol directly correlate with the occurrence of this disease while there seems to be somewhat more disagreement about the significance of the plasma concentration of triglycerides in this context.

In the recent decade it has been clearly shown that the concentrations of the various lipoproteins and their cholesterol and triglycerides content are of greater significance as risk factors for cardiovascular disease than are the total plasma levels of the lipids. Thus the amount of cholesterol in the Low Density Lipoprotein (LDL) and/or the Very Low Density Lipoproteins (VLDL) fractions is directly correlated to the risk for development of cardiovascular disease, while the cholesterol content in the most heavy fraction, High Density Lipoprotein (HDL), is indirectly correlated to the risk for vascular heart disease. We thus have 'bad cholesterol', e.g. the LDL- and/or the VLDL-cholesterol and 'good cholesterol', the HDL-cholesterol. Some type of ratio between these gives the most relevant description of the total cholesterol status of an individual.

The lipoproteins may be determined by various techniques such as electrophoresis, ultracentrifugation and precipitation. In the present study we assayed the HDL-cholesterol by precipitating the two light fractions and measuring the amount of cholesterol in the supernatant. We also determined the total concentration of cholesterol in the samples. Because of this technique we have expressed the ratio between the two types of cholesterol as the HDL-cholesterol/total cholesterol ratio. When an ultracentrifugation technique is employed this ratio is often given as the HDL-cholesterol/LDL-cholesterol or the inverse.

THE STUDY

The results of this investigation have been published elsewhere[1]. 98 women seeking contraceptive advice at the Department of

Obstetrics and Gynecology at the University of Linköping, Sweden, who gave their informed consent to participate in the study, were randomly allocated to 6 months of treatment with one of the four combinations of ethinyl estradiol (EE) and levonorgestrel (LNG) specified in Table 1. This table also gives the weight ratios between the estrogen and the progestogen in the four combinations. It varied from 0.08 (20/250) to 0.35 (Triquilar[R]).

Table 1 Composition of the four drugs used

Drug	*EE (μg)*	*LNG (μg)*	*EE/LNG ratio*
20/250	20	250	0.08
30/250	30	250	0.12
30/150	30	150	0.2
Triquilar[R]			
6 × 30/50 + 5 × 40/75 + 10 × 30/125			0.35

Fasting blood samples were obtained twice before treatment and after 1, 3 and 6 months of medication. In each blood sample the following lipid parameters were determined: total cholesterol, triglycerides, phospholipids, HDL-cholesterol and HDL-phospholipids. The SHBG capacity in the samples was determined by E. Johansson, Uppsala. All treatment results were compared to the mean of the two corresponding pretreatment values. The paired *t*-test was used for the statistical computations.

The results of the SHBG determinations are given in Figure 1 (Figures 1–6 are reproduced from *Fertilility and Sterility*, **35**, 172–179, 1981, after kind permission of American Fertility Society). It can be seen that the most estrogenic combination, Triquilar[R] (EE/LNG ratio = 0.35), raised this level considerably while on the other hand 20/250, the most progestogen-dominated drug (EE/LNG ratio = 0.08) induced a SHBG reduction of about 50%. The correlation between the changes of SHBG and the EE/LNG ratios was striking ($r = 0.977$).

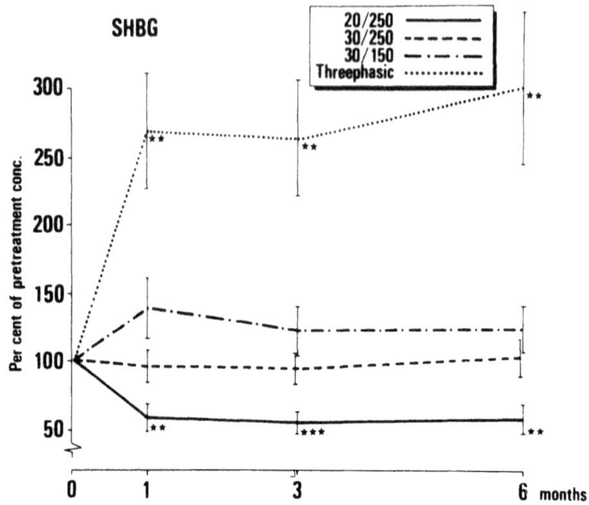

Figure 1 Effects of the four drugs on the plasma concentration of SHBG. The values are expressed as a mean percentage of the mean of the two pretreatment determinations. The bars show the standard errors of the mean. The significance of the mean differences was tested by paired *t*-tests and symbolized as follows: * $p < 0.05$; ** $p < 0.01$; *** $p < 0.001$ (From Larsson-Cohn, U., Fåhraeus, L., Wallentin, L. & Zador, G. (1981). Lipoprotein changes may be minimized by proper composition of a combined oral contraceptive. *Fertil. Steril.*, **35**, 172. Reproduced with the permission of the publisher, The American Fertility Society.)

It can thus be concluded that in the present dose range both SHBG and the EE/LNG ratio may be used as a crude index of the total estrogenicity of a combined oral contraceptive drug containing these two components.

Figure 2 demonstrates that all four drugs induced raised triglyceride levels although this was most noticeable among the women taking the triphasic drug (EE/LNG ratio = 0.35). This finding was not surprising as it is well established that estrogens raise triglycerides, possibly by inducing increased synthesis of the protein part of the VLDL particle. It is, however, noteworthy that none of the participants in any of the groups developed plasma triglyceride levels that were above what we consider as normal for females in this age group. Although increased triglycerides must be considered as an unwanted side-effect, it does not seem established if alterations of the magnitude found in this investigation may have any long-term clinical significance.

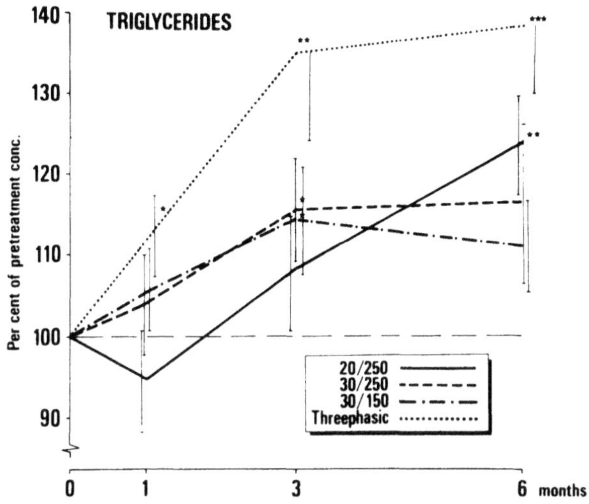

Figure 2 Effects of the four drugs on the plasma concentration of triglycerides. See also legend to Figure 1

The concentration of total cholesterol did not change dramatically during the period of treatment (Figure 3). This was in contrast to the levels of HDL-cholesterol (Figure 4). It can be seen that the triphasic drug was the only combination that did not have any significant effect on this parameter while the three others all induced lower concentrations. It should be observed that the HDL-cholesterol alterations appeared very rapidly. Already after the first treatment cycle all levels seemed to have been stabilized. The most noticeable reduction was shown by the women taking 20/250, e.g. the most progestogen-dominated drug (EE/LNG ratio = 0.08) while the changes in the 30/150 group (EE/LNG ratio = 0.2) were small. The combination

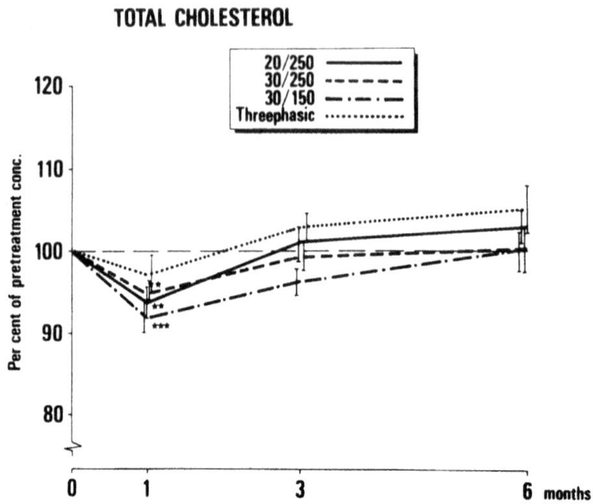

Figure 3 Effects of the four drugs on the plasma concentration of total cholesterol. See also legend to Figure 1

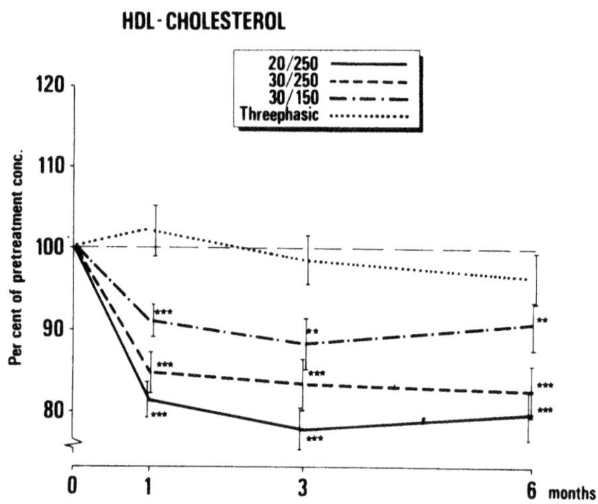

Figure 4 Effects of the four drugs on the plasma concentration of HDL-cholesterol. See also legend to Figure 1

30/250 came in between. It should be remarked that in a previous clinical investigation[2] with identical design 30/150 had no significant influence on the HDL-cholesterol levels. The possible reasons for this discrepancy in results were discussed in our original report[1].

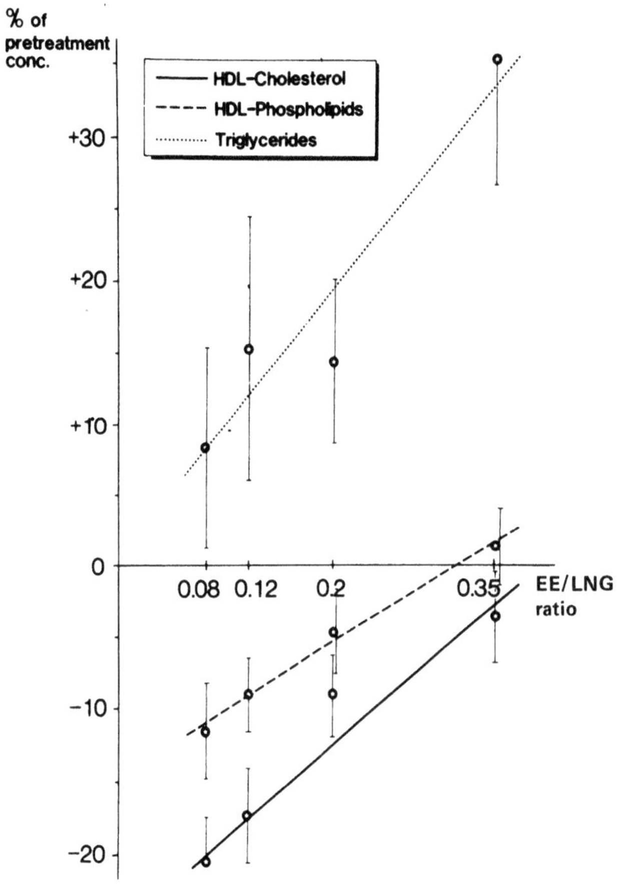

Figure 5 Correlations between the EE/LNG ratios and the 6 month changes in HDL-cholesterol (———) and HDL phospholipids (- - - - -) and the 3 month changes in triglycerides (· · · · · ·). See also legend to Figure 1

The coefficient of correlation between the changes of the HDL-cholesterol and EE/LNG ratios was 0.979 (unbroken line in Figure 5). Also the correlation between the changes of HDL-cholesterol and the changes of SHBG were good ($r = 0.915$). It thus seems that during combined oral contraceptive treatment the HDL-cholesterol varies according to the total estrogenicity of the given drug.

It was previously mentioned that some kind of ratio that takes into account both the 'good cholesterol' and the 'bad cholesterol'

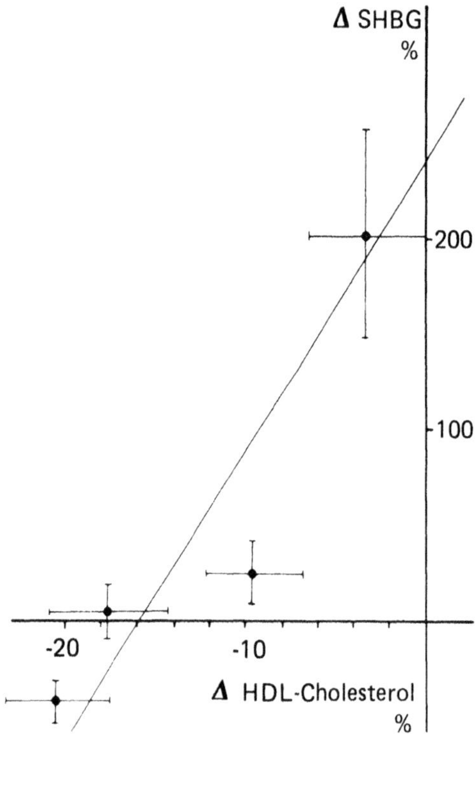

Figure 6 Correlation between the 6 month changes in SHBG and HDL-cholesterol. See also legend to Figure 1

probably gives the best estimate of an individual's total cholesterol status. Table 2 shows the changes of the mean HDL-cholesterol/total cholesterol ratios during this study. Both 20/250 and 30/250 induced a marked reduction down to levels that may be found in males with cardiovascular disease. The reduction that was seen in those on 30/150 and Triquilar was much lower and reached only a low level of statistical significance. It is noteworthy that the 6 months EE/LNG ratios in these two groups were in the same range as the pretreatment ratios of the two other combinations.

Table 2 **Effects of the four drugs in the HDL-cholesterol/total cholesterol ratio**

Drug	*Cycles of treatment*			
	0	*1*	*3*	*6*
20/250	0.32	0.28***	0.25***	0.25***
30/250	0.30	0.25***	0.26***	0.24***
30/150	0.35	0.34	0.32*	0.32*
Triquilar^R	0.33	0.34	0.31	0.31*

*$p < 0.05$
**$p < 0.01$
***$p < 0.001$

It can be concluded that our study has shown that it seems possible to minimize the lipoprotein alterations induced by EE/LNG combinations by carefully balancing the doses of the two components against each other.

References

1. Larsson-Cohn, U., Fåhraeus, L., Wallentin, L. and Zador, G. (1981). Lipoprotein changes may be minimized by proper composition of a combined oral contraceptive. *Fertil. Steril.*, **35**, 172
2. Larsson-Cohn, U., Wallentin, L. and Zador, G. (1979). Plasma lipids and high density lipoproteins during oral contraception with different combinations of ethinyl estradiol and levonorgestrel. *Horm. Metab. Res.*, **11**, 437

Chapter 10

Effects of a triphasic and a biphasic oral contraceptive on various hemostatic parameters

G. Winckelmann, E. Kaiser and H. L. Christl

There is general agreement that oral contraceptives may induce alterations in the hemostatic system resulting in a state of hypercoagulability[3-6,8,9]. Furthermore, it has been shown by some authors that the effect on the hemostatic system appears to depend mainly upon the dose of the estrogen component but also on the dose and type of the progestogen in the product used[1,2,7]. The clinical relevance of these changes occurring similarly and often more pronounced in pregnant women has, however, not been definitely proven.

The present paper presents the results of a double-blind study which was conducted to investigate the influence of a triphasic and a biphasic formulation of oral contraceptives on 12 selected hemostatic parameters.

MATERIALS AND METHODS

The triphasic contraceptive (T) contained 6 × 0.03 mg ethinyl estradiol (EE) + 0.05 mg levonorgestrel (LNG), 5 × 0.04 mg EE + 0.075 mg LNG and 10 × 0.03 mg EE + 0.125 mg LNG. The biphasic formulation (B) consisted of 7 × 0.05 mg ethinyl estradiol and 14 × 0.05 mg EE + 2.5 mg lynestrenol. Both contraceptives in uniform package were administered from the 5th to the 25–26th day of the cycles for 6 months.

Using random number tables, healthy women were assigned to one of the two different oral contraceptive formulations. 44 volunteers originally participated in the study. Eight women were excluded from the statistical evaluation for the following reasons: discontinuation of medication, simultaneous intake of other drugs, illness during the trial and laboratory tests not carried out in time. Finally, there were two equal groups of 18 each. Their age ranged from 19 to 40 years (mean 29.4) in one group (T) and from 22 to 44 years (mean 31.9) in the other one (B).

All laboratory tests were performed during the first phase (between days 4 and 6) and the second phase (between days 21 and 24) of the pretreatment cycle immediately before starting the intake of pills, of the second and sixth treatment cycle and of the second post-treatment cycle.

The following coagulation parameters were studied: platelet count, spontaneous platelet aggregation (photometric method), activated partial thromboplastin time, prothrombin time, anti-thrombin III (enzymatic determination using chromogenic substrates), fibrinogen, factor VII, factor VIII procoagulant activity (FVIII:C), factor VIII related antigen (FVIIIR:AG), factor VIII v. Willebrand factor activity (FVIIIR:vWF), fibrinogen–fibrin degradation products (by means of the staphylococcal clumping test) and fibrin monomer complexes (ethanol gelation test).

Data were statistically evaluated with analysis of variance for repeated measurements comparing the group mean values. If the results indicated differences during the trial course, a multiple comparative procedure (HSD-test according to Tukey) was subsequently applied.

RESULTS

In both trial groups most of the hemostatic parameters showed changes towards hypercoagulability during treatment with oral contraceptives. A positive ethanol gelation test indicating the appearance of fibrin monomer complexes was, however, found in one subject only. Fibrinogen–fibrin degradation products were slightly increased in three cases of each group in the second or sixth treatment cycle. Changes of all the other coagulation parameters affected most of the women to a variable degree.

Table 1 Changes of hemostatic parameters in the first (I) and second phase (II) of the 2nd and/or 6th cycles of treatment compared to the pretreatment cycle

	T		*B*	
	I	*II*	*I*	*II*
Platelet count	ns	+	+	+
Partial thromboplastin time	+	+	ns	+
Prothrombin time	ns	+	+	+

T = triphasic formulation; B = biphasic formulation.
+ statistically significant; ns not significant.

Table 2 Changes of hemostatic parameters in the first (I) and second phase (II) of the 2nd and/or 6th cycles of treatment compared to the pretreatment cycle

	T		*B*	
	I	*II*	*I*	*II*
Spontaneous platelet aggregation	+	ns	+	ns
Antithrombin III	ns	ns	ns	ns
Fibrinogen	+	+	ns	ns
Factor VII	+	+	+	+
Factor VIII:C	+	+	+	ns
Factor VIIIR:AG	ns	ns	ns	ns
Factor VIIIR:vWF	+	ns	+	+

T = triphasic formulation; B = biphasic formulation.
+ statistically significant; ns not significant.

The results of statistical evaluation are summarized in Tables 1 and 2. For most of the hemostatic parameters the differences between the mean values of the second and/or sixth treatment cycles and the pretreatment cycle were statistically significant at least on the 5% level. No significant difference in the changes of mean values was found between the two oral contraceptive groups. As a rule the coagulation parameters showed similar alterations during the first and second phase of cycles. Nevertheless a significant difference between the pretreatment and treatment values of a few coagulation factors was noted only in one of the two cycle phases which was most likely due to the considerable dispersion of the individual values. In this respect there were also some differences between the two oral contraceptive groups.

The most strongly affected coagulation factors were factor VII, v.Willebrand factor and factor VIII procoagulant activity. The changes in factor VII and v.Willebrand factor are presented in Figures 1 and 2. The results are expressed as percentages of mean values in the pretreatment cycles.

Maximum changes for most of the coagulation factors had already occurred in the second treatment cycle. Afterwards the mean values of some parameters (AT III, fibrinogen, FVIIIR:vWF, FVIIIR:AG, aPTT) in both trial groups moved towards the pretreatment values again (see changes in fibrinogen levels and antithrombin III, Figures 3 and 4).

It should be stressed at this point that the mean values of all hemostatic parameters always remained within the normal range during treatment with oral contraceptives, even when their changes were statistically significant. Also the individual values of the great majority of the women did not exceed the normal range. However, there were some individuals in both groups who, sometimes repeatedly, showed abnormal values in several coagulation parameters (see Figures 5 and 6). In this respect somewhat more pathological changes in some coagulation factors seemed to occur in the subjects receiving the biphasic formulation than in those who took the triphasic contraceptive.

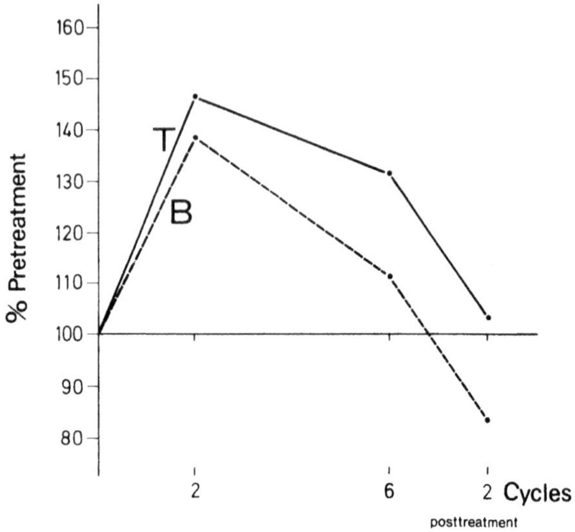

(a)

(1st Phase of Cycles)

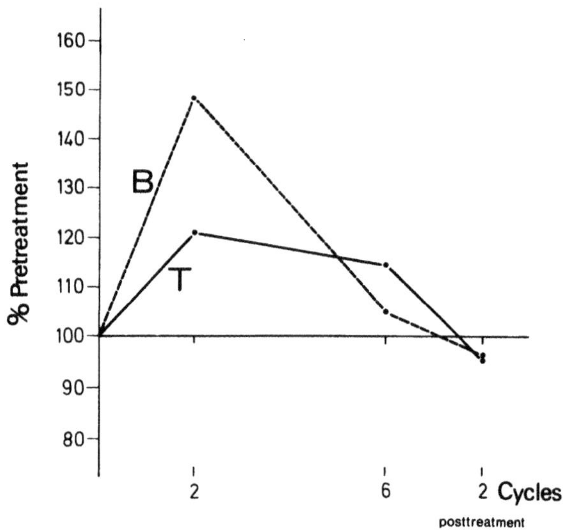

(b)

(2nd Phase of Cycles)

Figures 1(a),(b) Changes in factor VII in the first (a) and a second phase (b) of cycles during and after treatment with oral contraception. Means expressed as percentage pretreatment values. T = Triphasic product; B = Biphasic product

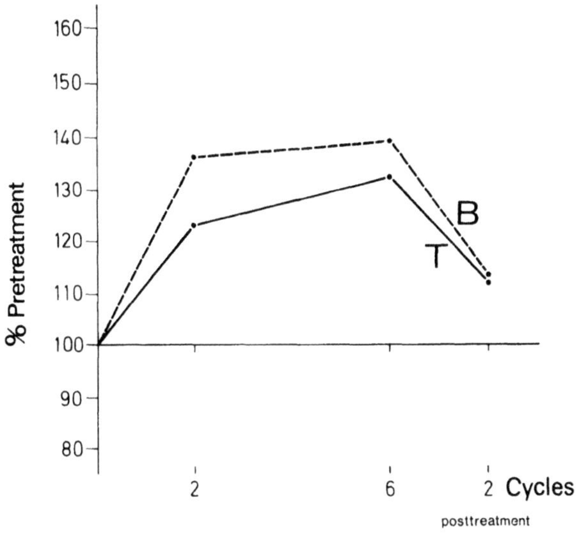

(a)

(1st Phase of Cycles)

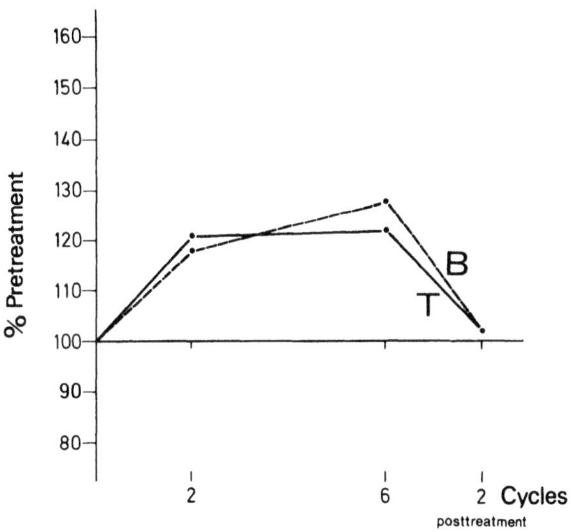

(b)

(2nd Phase of Cycles).

Figures 2(a),(b) Changes in factor VIII v.Willebrand activity (FVIIIR: vWF) in the first (a) and second phase (b) of cycles during and after treatment with oral contraception. Means expressed as percentage of the pretreatment values. T = Triphasic product; B = Biphasic product

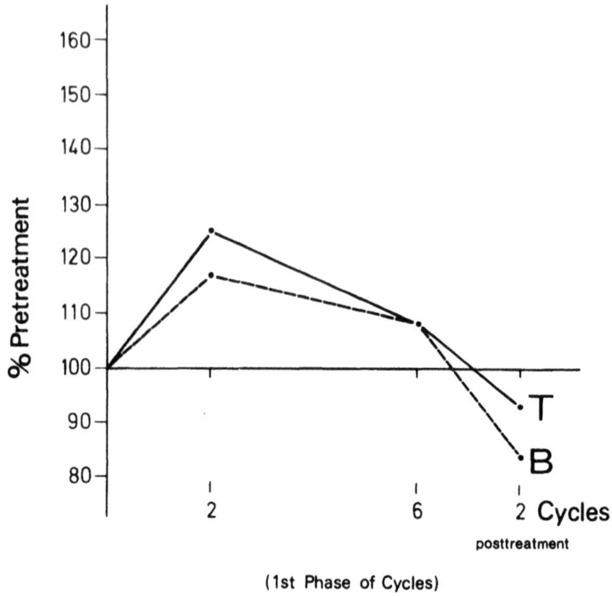

Figure 3 Changes in fibrinogen in the first phase of cycles during and after treatment with oral contraception. Means expressed as percentage of the pretreatment values. T = Triphasic product; B = Biphasic product

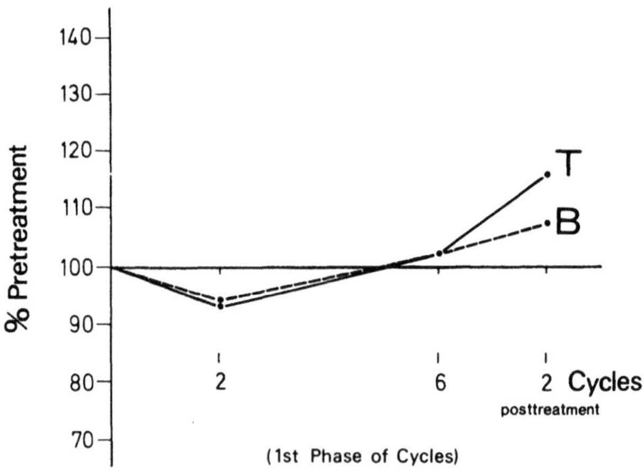

Figure 4 Changes in antithrombin III in the first phase of cycles during and after treatment with oral contraception. Means expressed as percentage of the pretreatment values. T = Triphasic product; B = Biphasic product

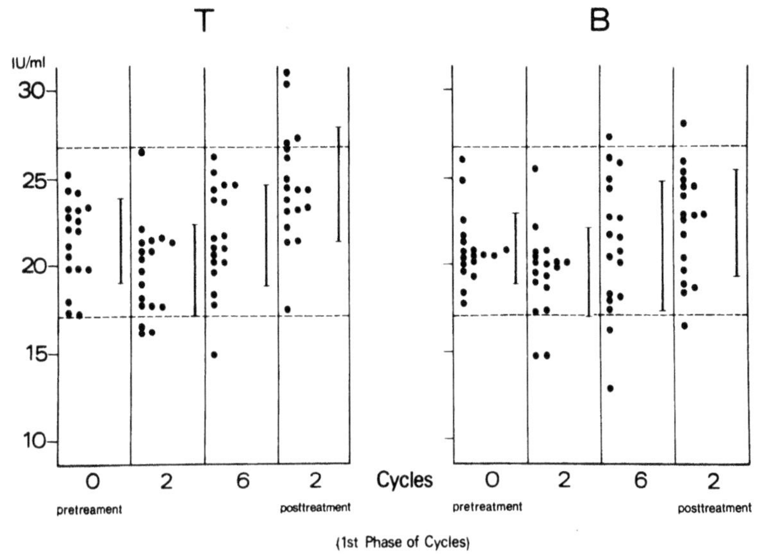

Figure 5 Individual values of antithrombin III before, during and after treatment with oral contraception. T = Triphasic product; B = Biphasic product

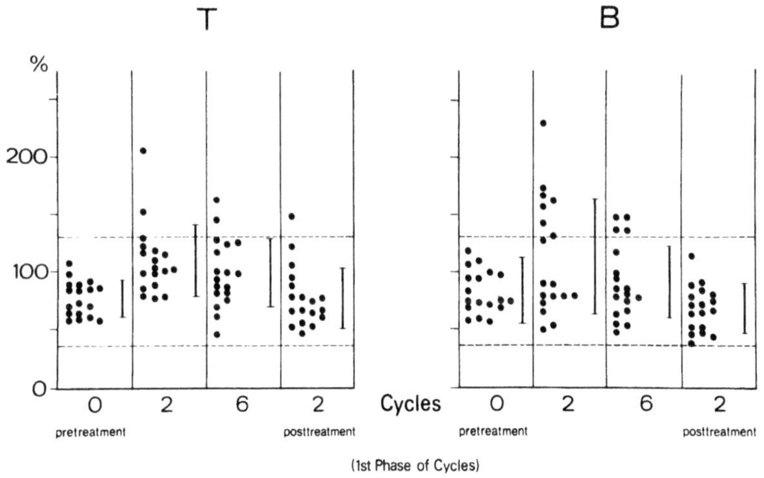

Figure 6 Individual values of factor VIII v.Willebrand activity (FVIIIR: vWF) before, during and after treatment with oral contraception. T = Triphasic product; B = Biphasic product

COMMENT

Assuming that alterations of the hemostatic system induced by oral contraceptives are of importance for the development of thromboembolic complications, one should expect that changes within the normal range even when statistically very significant are not of clinical relevance, but rather those which result in pathological values of the hemostatic parameters during treatment. The risk of thromboembolism is supposed to be the greater, the more procoagulants will be increased and the more physiological inhibitors as well as the fibrinolytic potential will be depressed.

Taking six selected hemostatic parameters as a basis we analysed how many of them became abnormal during oral contraceptive treatment in each patient. The parameters selected were spontaneous platelet aggregation, antithrombin III, fibrinogen, factor VII, FVIII:C and FVIIIR:vWF. As shown in Table 3 only a few of these parameters were found to be pathological in the majority of the women, while in some cases four or even five of the selected six hemostatic factors were affected. The hemostatic system of these latter subjects apparently tends to react more heavily to the oral contraceptive tested by an increased coagulability.

Table 3 Number of subjects with pathological findings of six selected hemostatic parameters during oral contraceptive treatment

No. of tests with pathological results	*No. of subjects*
0	5
+	10
+ +	13
+ + +	5
+ + + +	2
+ + + + +	1

Hemostatic parameters: Spontaneous platelet aggregation, Antithrombin III, Fibrinogen, Factor VII, Factor VIII:C, Factor VIIIR:vWF.

From our observations, one may conclude that changes in the hemostatic system induced by oral contraceptives do not only depend on the product formulation but also on the individual response which seems to be higher in some women than in the majority of oral contraceptive users.

SUMMARY

Changes in 12 selected blood coagulation parameters were studied in a double-blind trial in 36 women receiving one of two formulations of oral contraceptives over 6 months. The oral contraceptives used were a triphasic formulation of ethinyl estradiol (0.03 – 0.04 – 0.03 mg) + levonorgestrel (0.05 – 0.075 – 0.125 mg) and a biphasic formulation of ethinyl estradiol (0.05 mg) and ethinyl estradiol (0.05 mg) + lynestrenol (2.5 mg). The laboratory tests were performed during the first and second phase of the pretreatment cycle, the second and sixth treatment cycle and the second post-treatment cycle. Mean values of almost all coagulation parameters showed changes consistent with hypercoagulability, at least during the second treatment cycle in both groups. The differences between the pretreatment and treatment values were statistically significant for the following parameters in both groups: spontaneous platelet aggregation, fibrinogen, factor VII, factor VIII procoagulant activity, factor VIII v.Willebrand factor, activated partial thromboplastin time, prothrombin time and platelet counts. All mean treatment values remained within the normal range and no significant difference was found between the two oral contraceptive groups. There were, however, certain individuals in both groups who showed abnormal values in several coagulation parameters indicating an increased response of their hemostatic system to the oral contraceptive tested. Changes in coagulation parameters induced by oral contraception thus appear not only to depend on the product formulation but also on the individual response which seems to be higher in some women than in the majority of oral contraceptive users.

References

1. Briggs, M. and Briggs, M. (1980). A randomized study of metabolic effects of four oral contraceptive preparations containing levonorgestrel plus ethinyloestradiol in different regimens. In Greenblatt, R. B. (ed.) *The Development of a New Triphasic Oral Contraceptive.* pp. 79–98. (Lancaster: MTP Press)
2. Conrad, J., Samama, M. and Salomon, Y. (1972). Antithrombin III and the oestrogen content of combined oestro-progestagen contraceptives. *Lancet*, **2**, 1148
3. Dugdale, M. and Masi, A. T. (1971). Hormonal contraception and thromboembolic diseases: effects of the oral contraceptives on hemostatic mechanisms. A review of the literature. *J. Chronic Dis.*, **23**, 775
4. Hedlin, A. M. (1975). The effect of oral contraceptive estrogen on blood coagulation and fibrinolysis. *Thromb. Diathes. Haemorrh. (Stuttg.)* **33**, 370
5. von Kaulla, E., Droegemueller, W., Aoki, N. and von Kaulla, K. N. (1971). Antithrombin III depression and thrombin generation acceleration in woman taking oral contraceptives. *Am. J. Obstet. Gynecol.*, **109**, 868
6. Ludwig, H. (1970). Ovulationshemmer, Hämostase und Gefäßkomplikationen. *Der Gynäkologe*, **2**, 195
7. Meade, T. W., Haines, A. P., North, W. R. S., Chakrabarti, R., Howarth, D. J. and Stirling, Y. (1977). Haemostatic, lipid, and blood-pressure profiles of women on oral contraceptives containing 50 μg or 30 μg oestrogen. *Lancet*, **2**, 948
8. Poller, L. (1978). Oral contraceptives, blood clotting and thrombosis. *Br. Med. Bull.*, **34**, 151
9. Roy, S., Mishell, D. R., Gray, G., Dozono-Takano, R., Brenner, P. F., Eide, I., de Quattro, V. and Shaw, S. T. (1980). Comparison of metabolic and clinical effects of four oral contraceptive formulations and a contraceptive vaginal ring. *Am. J. Obstet. Gynecol.*, **136**, 920

Chapter 11

Comparative investigation of oral contraceptives using randomized, prospective protocols

M. H. Briggs

INTRODUCTION

Combined oral contraceptives, containing a synthetic estrogen and a synthetic progestogen, have been in worldwide use for more than a generation. While only two estrogens (ethinyl estradiol and mestranol) have been used in commercial formulations, at least 14 different progestogens have been tried[1]. Large epidemiological surveys of oral contraceptive users have suggested that some of the adverse clinical associations of oral contraception are related to the daily estrogen dose, though others are related to the daily progestogen dose[2]. In an attempt to produce safer and more acceptable preparations, manufacturers have introduced a range of low dose oral contraceptive formulations. Particular attention has been placed on the estrogen component and most of these new formulations contain a daily dose of 30 or 35 μg estrogen. Epidemiological evidence suggests that these low estrogen formulations have indeed reduced the incidence of some rare, but serious, side-effects of oral contraception[3,4]. Recently a new progestogen (desogestrel, ORG 2969) has also been introduced and claimed to have a more favorable impact on laboratory indices of cardiovascular risk[5]. The present study was undertaken to compare the metabolic impact of several different oral contraceptive formulations on young, healthy, new oral contraceptive acceptors.

METHODS AND MATERIALS

Study No. 1

The four products investigated were all commercial formulations containing the same estrogen (EE) and progestogen (LNG). They were:

2 monophasic	(× 21)	0.150 mg LNG + 30 μg EE
	(× 21)	0.250 mg LNG + 50 μg EE
1 biphasic	(× 10)	0.050 mg LNG + 50 μg EE
	(× 11)	0.125 mg LNG + 50 μg EE
1 triphasic	(× 6)	0.050 mg LNG + 30 μg EE
	(× 5)	0.075 mg LNG + 40 μg EE
	(× 10)	0.125 mg LNG + 30 μg EE

Criteria to enter the study included an absence of any absolute or relative contraindication to hormonal contraception, a body weight within ± 10% of the ideal for height, no concurrent medication, normotension, good personal motivation, age less than 30 years, and non-use of cigarettes.

During the immediate pretreatment cycle, the women used a barrier contraceptive: oral contraception was started on day 5 of the first treatment cycle.

Blood specimens were collected from the antecubital vein of subjects who had fasted overnight. Two specimens were taken on consecutive days during the late pretreatment cycle (days 25–28) and during each treatment cycle on either of the last 2 days of pill taking.

An oral glucose tolerance test and measurements of the renin-angiotensin system were conducted during the immediate pretreatment cycle and again every six cycles. Blood coagulation and fibrinolytic factors (fibrinogen, factor VII, factor VIII, factor X, plasminogen, antithrombin III) were measured every three cycles. Fasting plasma lipids (total cholesterol, HDL-cholesterol, triglycerides) were measured each cycle. References to laboratory methods are given in detail elsewhere[6].

RESULTS

Study No. 1

The data reported in the present paper summarizes results after 18 treatment cycles. Previous publications[6-8] have reported results after 6, 9 and 12 cycles respectively. Up to 12 cycles, results on women who discontinued were excluded, so that all the data up to that time are for the same 91 individuals, approximately equally divided between the four groups. After the 12th cycle there were further dropouts (almost entirely for non-medical reasons). The results from 12 to 18 cycles include those women remaining in the study (85 by 18 cycles). Exclusion of the six dropouts did not affect significantly the mean results for any parameter at earlier results.

Mean results for each group in oral glucose tolerance tests are shown in Figure 1, which gives results at cycles 0, 6 and 12. Mean plasma insulin responses during these tests are also shown. A similar test was conducted towards the end of cycle-18, but as there was no significant difference between the results at cycles 12 and 18, for either glucose or insulin, these have not been added to Figure 1.

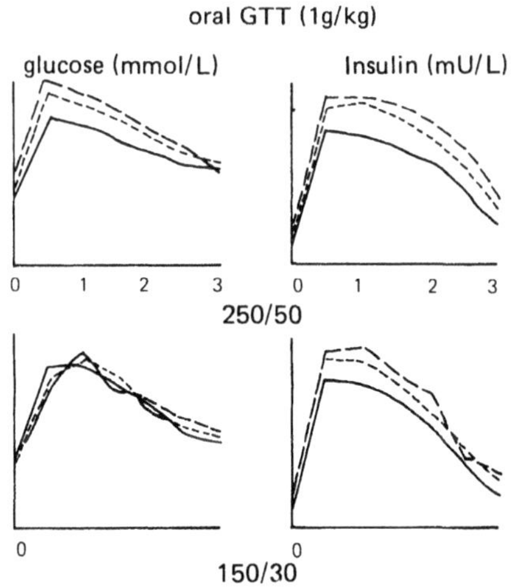

Figure 1
(Part 1)

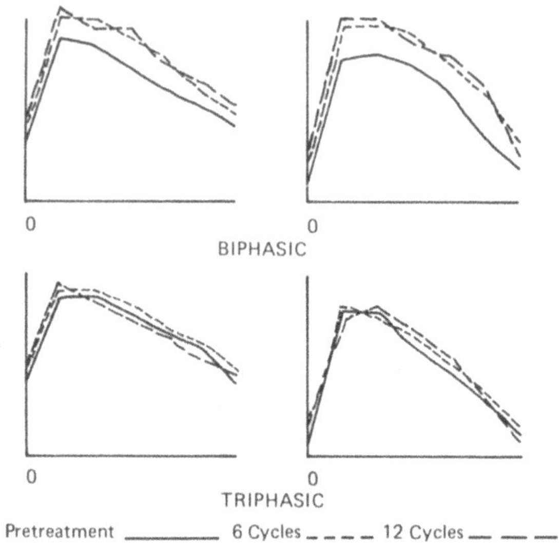

Figure 1 Oral glucose tolerance tests (1 g/kg) and plasma insulin responses

Figures 2–4 (below). *Changes in fasting lipids in volunteers assigned at random to four different combined oral contraceptives. Key: see p. 116*

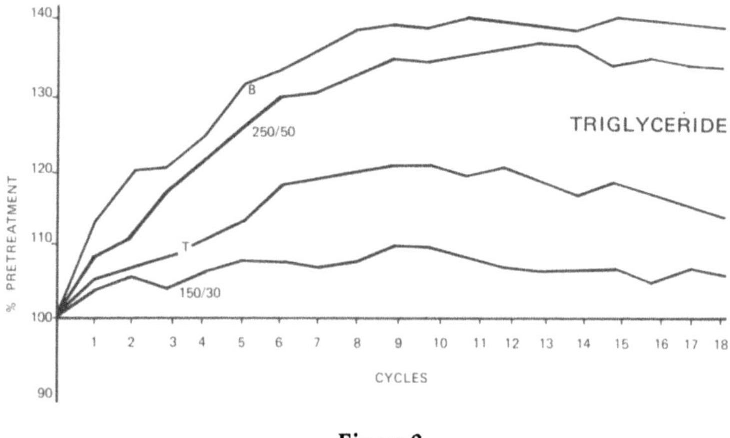

Figure 2

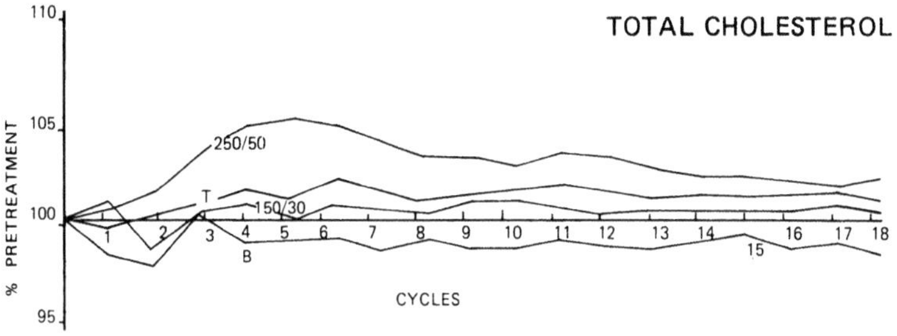

Figure 3

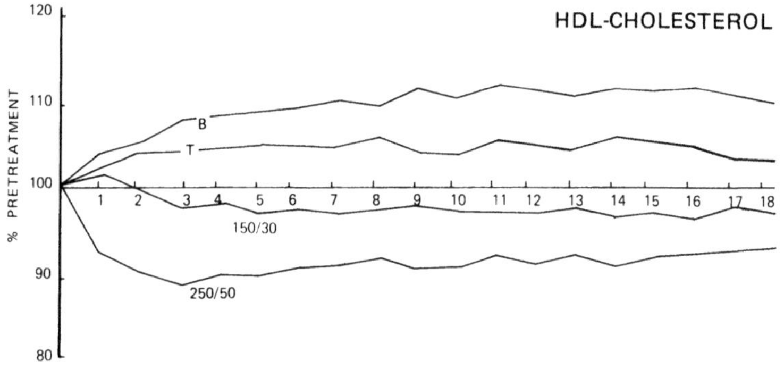

Figure 4

Figures 5–10 (below). *Changes in blood coagulation factors and related parameters in volunteers assigned at random to four different oral contraceptives. Key: see p. 116*

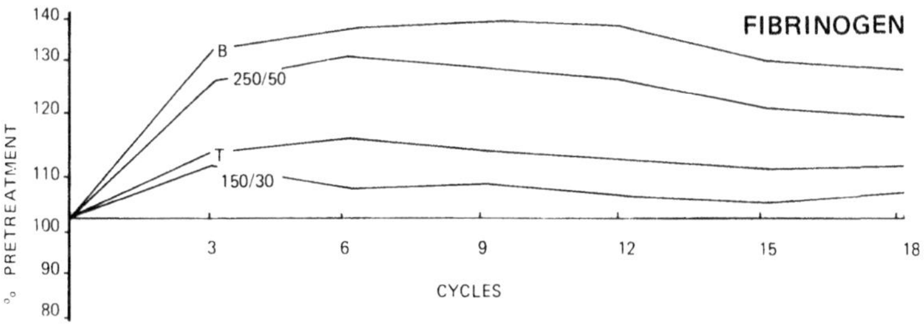

Figure 5

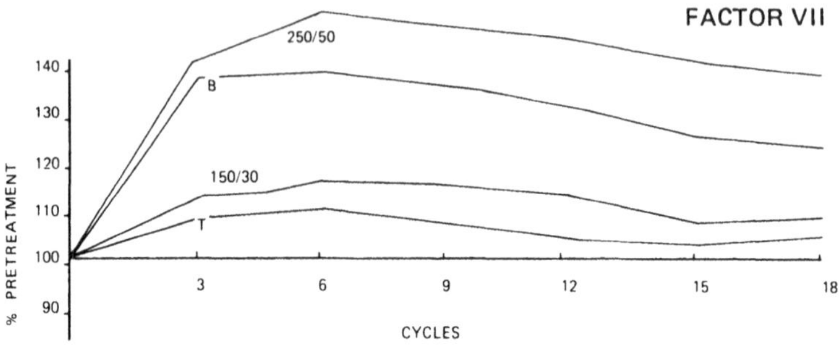

Figure 6

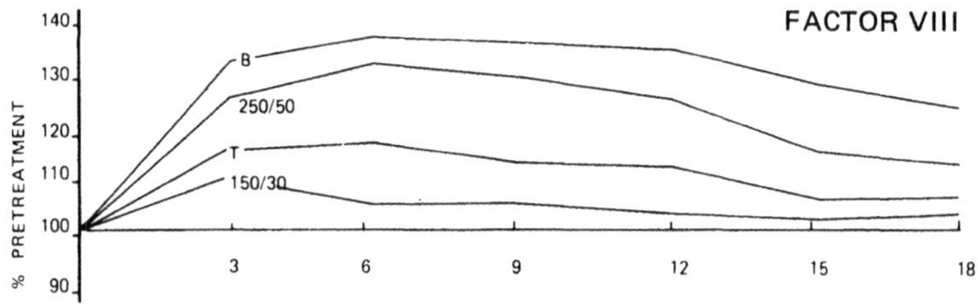

Figure 7

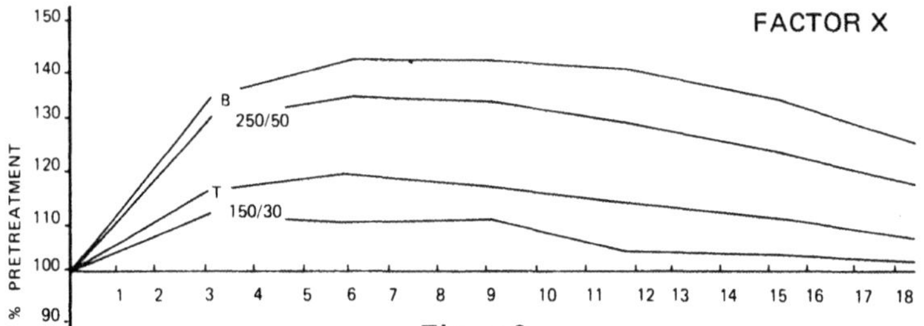

Figure 8

The monthly variations in mean concentrations of triglycerides, total and HDL-cholesterol in fasting plasma are shown respectively in Figures 2–4. Fibrinogen and coagulation factors VII, VIII, and X, together with the fibrinolytic factors plasminogen and antithrombin III, all of which were determined every three cycles, are presented as mean values for each group in Figures 5–10. Results are percentages of values in the pretreatment cycles.

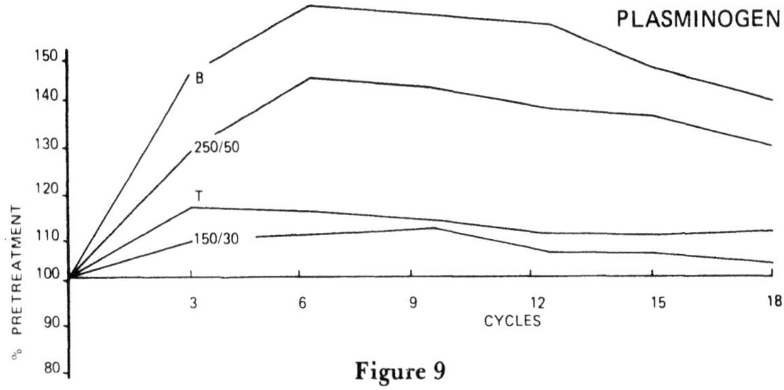

Figure 9

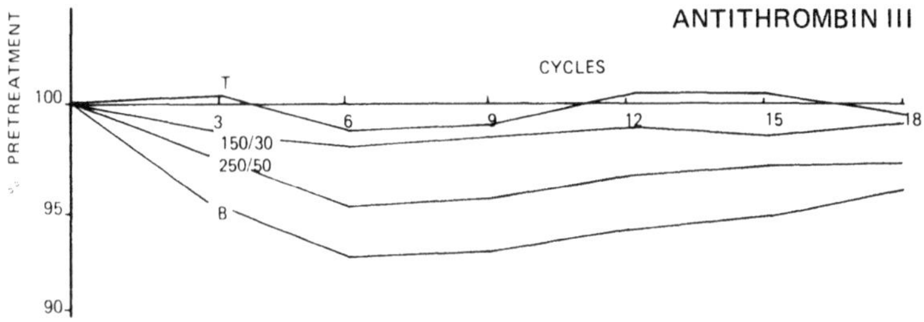

Figure 10

Mean values for renin-substrate concentration, renin activity, and renin concentration, measured every 6 months, are plotted in Figure 11.

DISCUSSION

Study No. 1

It is apparent that combined oral contraception based on LNG and EE induces statistically significant changes in a number of important metabolic parameters. These changes are established by the end of the first treatment cycle, but their magnitude depends on formulation. Significant further variations also occur depending upon the duration of treatment.

For the oral GTT curves, significant deterioration occurs at 6, 12 and 18 cycles for the 250/50 and biphasic formulations, but not for the 150/30 or triphasic preparations. This suggests that the estrogen dose is of major importance for this change. Inter-

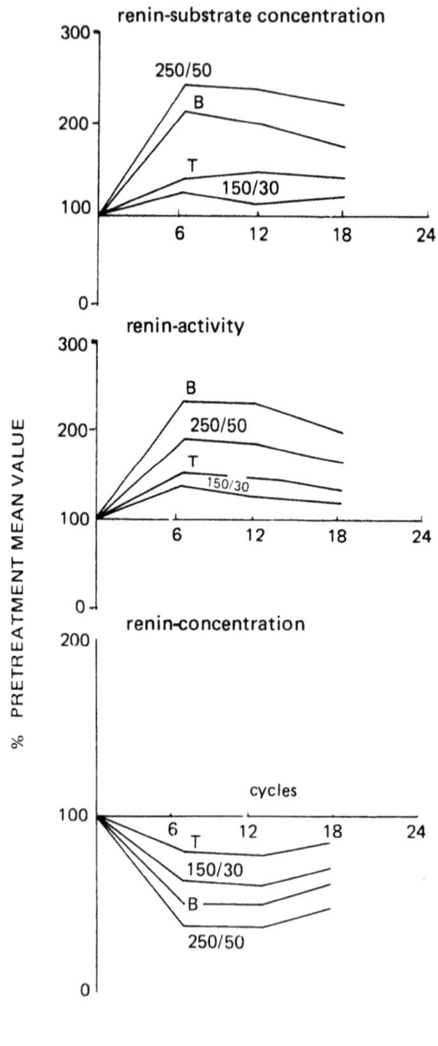

Figure 11 Changes in plasma renin-angiotensin system

pretation of the plasma insulin response, however, is more complex. Of the four products, only the triphasic formulation is without significant effect, so that the progestogen dose may be important in determining this change, with positive synergism between the two hormones being a further factor.

Significant increases in fasting triglycerides occur with all formulations, though those with 150/30 (+5–6%) and the triphasic (+12–18%) were much less than for the biphasic (+30–35%) and 250/50 (+35–38%) formulations.

Interestingly, fasting triglyceride concentration continues to rise for up to nine treatment cycles, then plateaus, though some decline in mean values appears to occur in the final few cycles.

There were few changes in total cholesterol, though a small (+5%) but significant increase occurred with the 250/50 formulation. As the change with the biphasic product, which has the same estrogen dose, was quite different, it is likely that the progestogen component alone is of major importance. Quite different effects are seen for HDL-cholesterol, where the major increase is with the biphasic product, and the largest mean decrease with 250/50.

There is good evidence from several studies[9–12] that HDL-cholesterol is elevated by estrogens, but suppressed by progestogens and androgens. This is clearly seen in the present results, where the maximum increase is with a high estrogen, low progestogen product, while the highest dose progestogen formulation leads to the greatest drop.

The antiestrogenic effect of LNG is also seen in results for the various coagulation factors. These are well known to be stimulated by estrogens[13], while the antagonistic effect of progestogens simultaneously administered has been documented by several people[14,15]. Most factors show similar changes, with the two highest dose estrogen formulations producing the greatest increases. For all factors except VII (where the results are anomalous), the increase with 250/50 (which has the largest progestogen dose) is less than for the biphasic formulation. Similarly, the increases with 150/30 are less than for the triphasic (again except for factor VII).

Maximum increases for coagulation factors occur by about treatment cycle 6, remain constant until cycle 12, then show a significant decrease towards the pretreatment mean values for each group.

Plasminogen shows a similar response to the coagulation factors, together with a tendency to return towards the pretreatment values in the later cycles. Antithrombin III, however, is suppressed to variable extents during oral contraceptive use. The greatest effect is with the biphasic product, which suggests an estrogenic effect. As the response with 250/50 is also significant, but less than for biphasic, the progestogen appears to be antagonistic. Changes with 150/30 and the triphasic formulation were not statistically significant.

The final parameters examined in this study of four formulations were concerned with the renin-angiotensin system. There is significant increase in the renin-substrate concentration, with the rise following use of 250/50 being greater than that with the biphasic formulation. Changes with the triphasic and 150/30 preparations were much less. Renin activity is also significantly raised, with maximum increases being seen with the biphasic, followed by 250/50. The expected suppression in renin concentration is approximately in proportion to the rise in renin-substrate.

As with the various coagulation factors, the changes in renin-angiotensin parameters were maximal at cycles 6–12, but they tended to return towards pretreatment mean values by cycle 18.

METHODS AND MATERIALS

Study No. 2

This was conducted to the same protocol as the first study, except that the three products used were:

1 monophasic	(× 21) 0.150 mg DOG	+	30 μg EE
1 biphasic	(× 7)		50 μg EE
	(× 15) 0.125 mg DOG	+	50 μg EE
1 triphasic	(× 6) 0.050 mg LNG	+	30 μg EE
	(× 5) 0.075 mg LNG	+	40 μg EE
	(× 10) 0.125 mg LNG	+	30 μg EE

EE = ethinyl estradiol; LNG = levonorgestrel,
DOG = desogestrel

RESULTS

Study No. 2

At the time of preparing this report, 31 women had completed four treatment cycles. Of these, 11 were receiving the monophasic product, 11 the biphasic, and 9 the triphasic. Pretreatment glucose tolerance tests have been conducted, together with measurements of the renin system. These will be repeated at the end of cycle 6.

Monthly results for fasting plasma triglycerides, total cholesterol and HDL-cholesterol are shown in Figures 12–14. Changes in coagulation and fibrinolytic factors are in Figures 15–20. Again all results are shown as means and as percentages of values in the pretreatment cycles.

DISCUSSION

The second study has only been in progress for four* treatment cycles and biochemical changes are limited; nevertheless some significant differences between the three products are already apparent. The biphasic† formulation shows considerable effects on triglycerides (+30%), whereas the monophasic† and

*At the time of going to press figures were updated to six cycles.

†Note that these formulations contain DOG and are different to the monophasic and biphasic formulations of Study No. 1

Figures 12–14 (below). *Changes in fasting plasma lipids in 31 young women assigned at random to three different oral contraceptive preparations.* *Key: see p. 124*

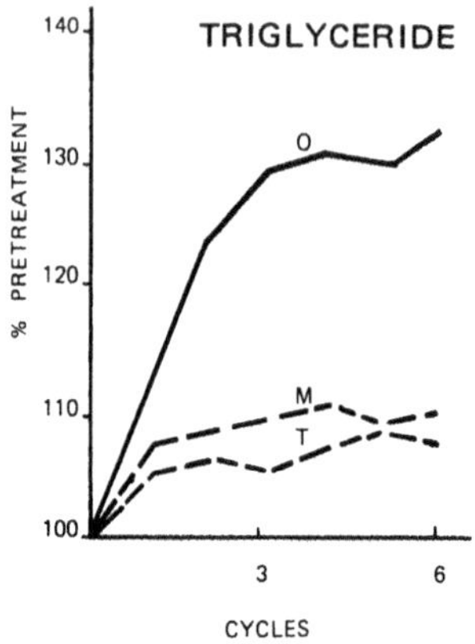

Figure 12

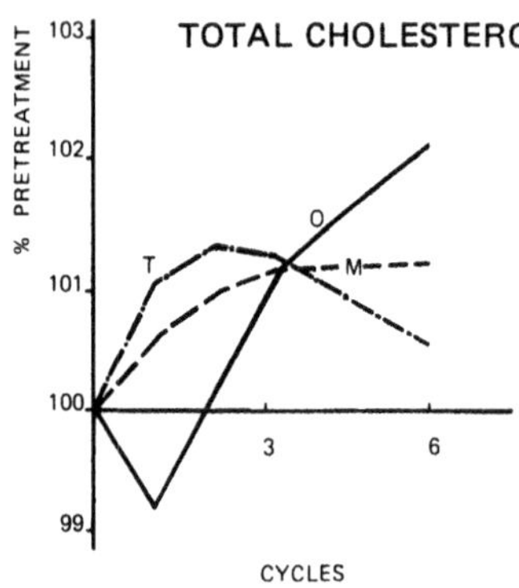

Figure 13

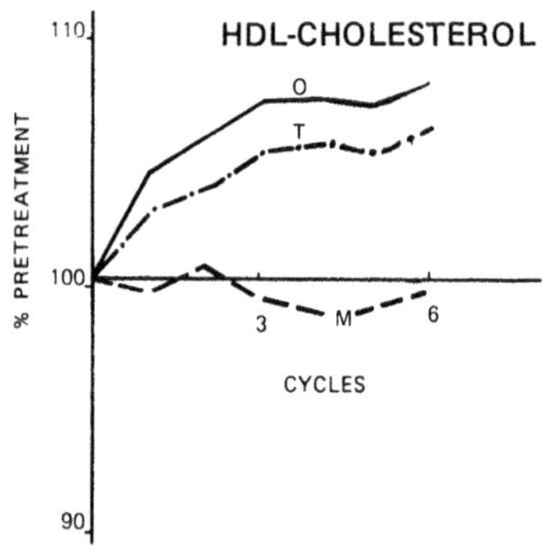

Figure 14

Figures 15–20 (below). *Changes in blood coagulation factors and related parameters in 31 young women assigned at random to three different oral contraceptive preparations. Key: see p. 124*

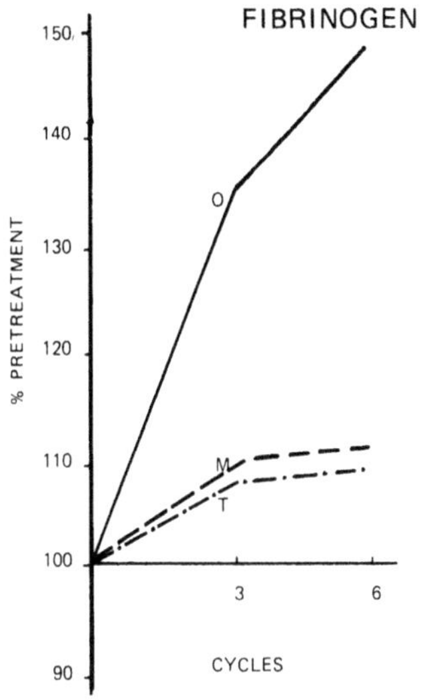

Figure 15

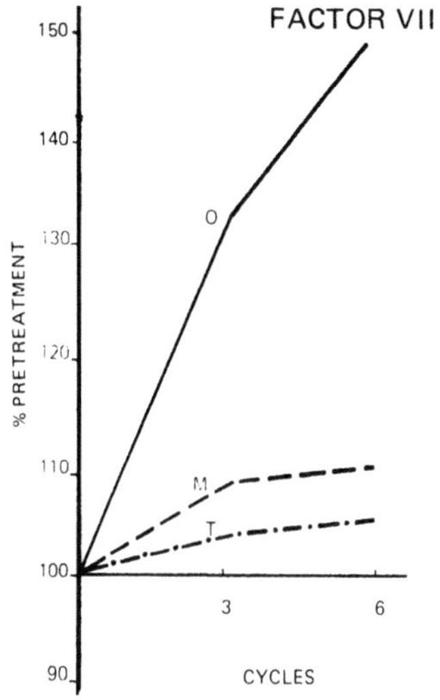

Figure 16

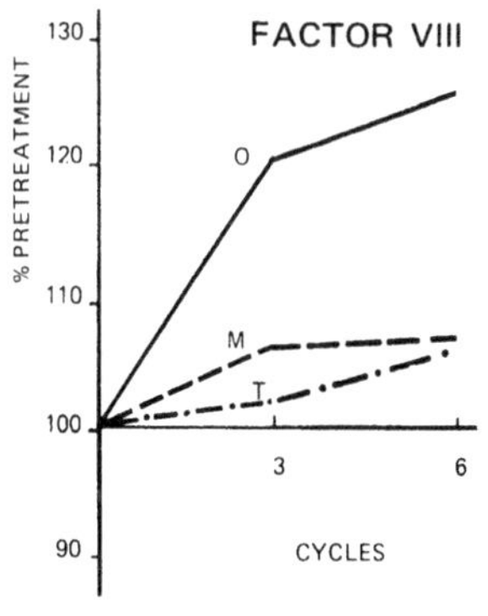

Figure 17

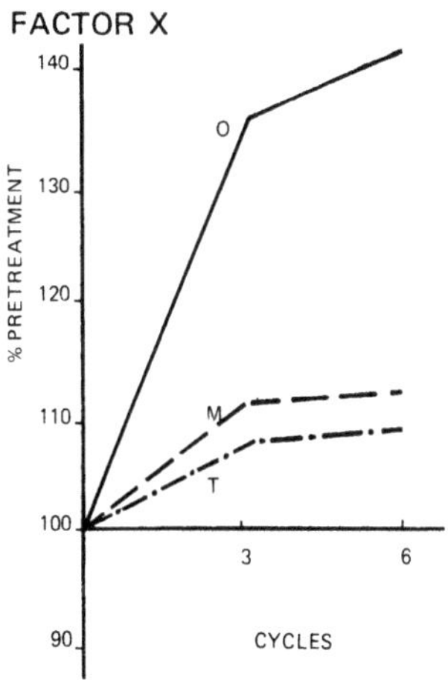

Figure 18

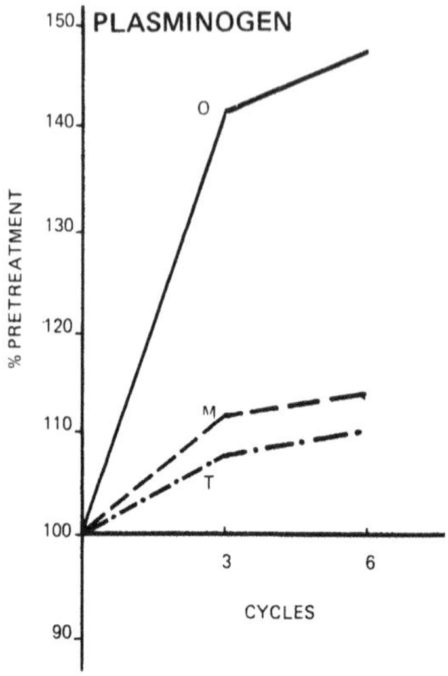

Figure 19

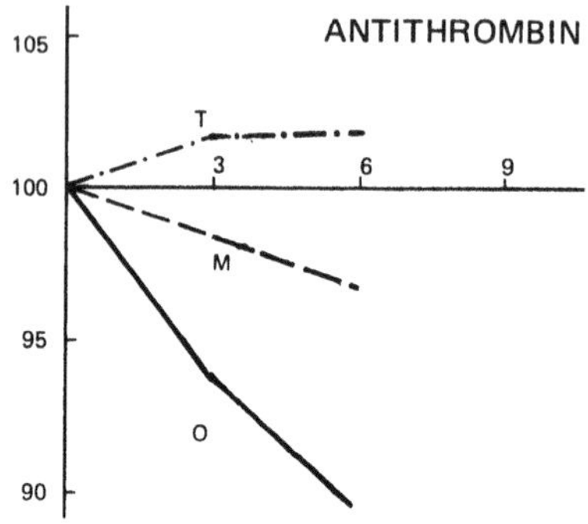

Figure 20

triphasic formulations produce much smaller (+ 8–10%) mean changes. For HDL-cholesterol the biphasic† showed an increase similar to the triphasic, while the monophasic† was associated with a small decrease over pretreatment values.

Significant increases are seen in many coagulation factors during the use of all three products, but the changes with the biphasic formulation are very much greater than with the other two. Similarly, antithrombin III is significantly suppressed by the biphasic, but not by the others.

CONCLUSIONS

(1) Significant alterations occur in biochemical parameters (GTT, plasma lipids, coagulation factors, renin-angiotensin system) related to cardiovascular disease risks in many women using oral contraceptives. These alterations are significantly affected by the product formulation, with maximum metabolic impact resulting from use of high doses of both estrogen and progestogen.

Minimum changes were seen in women receiving low dose, fixed (150/30) or triphasic preparations of levonorgestrel with EE.

(2) Changes in some biochemical parameters were established over 3–6 treatment cycles (e.g. HDL-cholesterol), but others (e.g. triglycerides) did not peak until cycles 9–12. Some of the changes (e.g. in coagulation factors and the renin-angiotensin system) showed a significant trend to return to pretreatment values after 12 cycles.

(3) In terms of biochemical impact on cardiovascular risk factors, the new progestogen desogestrel appears to offer no advantage over the well-established levonorgestrel.

References

1. Briggs, M. H. (1977). Combined oral contraceptives. In Diczfalusy, E. (ed.) *Regulation of Human Fertility*. pp. 253–282. (Copenhagen: Scriptor)
2. Royal College of General Practitioners (1974). *Oral Contraceptives and Health*. (London: Pitman)
3. Meade, T. W., Greenberg, G. and Thompson, S. C. (1980). Progestogens and cardiovascular reactions associated with oral contraceptives and a comparison of the safety of 50 and 30 μg estrogen preparations. *Br. Med. J.* **1**, 1157
4. Böttiger, L. E., Boman, G., Eklund, G. and Westerholm, B. (1980). Oral contraceptives and thromboembolic disease: effects of lowering oestrogen content. *Lancet*, **1**, 1097
5. Bergink, E. W., Hamburger, A. D., de Jayer, E. and Van der Vies, J. (1981). Binding of a contraceptive progestogen ORG 2969 and its metabolites to receptor proteins and human sex hormone binding globulin. *J. Steroid Biochem.*, **14**, 175
6. Briggs, M. H. and Briggs, M. (1980). A randomized study of metabolic effects of four oral contraceptive preparations containing laevonorgestrel plus ethinyloestradiol in different regimens. *Reproduccion*, **4**, suppl. 79
7. Briggs, M. H. (1980). Metabolic effects of the pill. *Bull. Postgrad. Committee Med., Univ. Sydney*, **36**, 148
8. Briggs, M. H. and Briggs, M. (1981) Randomized prospective studies on metabolic effects of oral contraceptives. *Acta Obstet. Gynecol. Scand. Suppl. 105, 25*

9. Krauss, R. M., Lindgren, F. T., Wingerd, J., Bradley, D. D. and Ramcharan, S. (1979). Effect of estrogens and progestins on high density lipoproteins. *Lipids*, **14**, 113
10. Briggs, M. H. and Briggs, M. (1979). Plasma lipoprotein changes during oral contraception. *Curr. Med. Res. Opin.*, **6**, 249
11. Larsson-Cohn, U., Faaraeus, L., Wallentin, L. and Zador, G. (1981). Lipoprotein changes may be minimised by proper composition of a combined oral contraceptive. *Fertil. Steril.*, **35**, 172
12. Bradley, D. D., Wingerd, J., Petitti, D. B., Krauss, R. M. and Ramcharan, S. (1978). Serum high-density lipoprotein cholesterol in women using oral contraceptives, estrogens and progestins. *N. Engl. Med. J.*, **299**, 17
13. Poller, L. (1978). Oral contraceptives, blood clotting, and thrombosis. *Br. Med. Bull.*, **34**, 151
14. Briggs, M. H. (1974). Thromboembolism and oral contraceptives. *Br. Med. J.*, **2**, 503
15. Sabra, A. M. A. and Bonnar, J. (1979). Comparable effects of 30 and 50 μg oestrogen-progestogen oral contraceptives and blood clotting and fibrinolysis. *Thrombosis Haemostasis*, **42**, 25

Discussion

Question Dr Larsson-Cohn's trial shows a change in HDL depending on the ethinyl estradiol/levonorgestrel ratio. Users of the triphasic formulation have experience of three different ratios in each cycle. When did you take the blood samples?

Dr Larsson-Cohn The samples were taken on the last and second last day of the treatment period. We have not assessed the changes during the cycle but the halflife of HDL is not all that short and thus any alteration during the cycle would not be large.

Question If the HDL/total cholesterol ratio is favorable, and dependent therefore on a high ethinyl estradiol/norgestrel ratio, should we have preference for a 50 μg monophasic pill instead of a 30 μg – from the view of preventing atherosclerosis?

Dr Larsson-Cohn From the pure HDL/cholesterol view I would query that. With the same dose of progestogen a moderate increase of ethinyl estradiol may be favorable.

Question Could the difference in ischemic heart disease incidence between men and women be that men have more stress?

Dr Larsson-Cohn Ischemic heart disease is, of course, a multifactorial disease.

Question How can you explain the fact that the increase in triglycerides in triphasic users as found by Dr Larsson-Cohn is much higher than that found by Professor Briggs?

Dr Larsson-Cohn I have no explanation – but we all work with small groups and random changes must be expected.

Question Does Dr Winckelmann believe that patients with very low antithrombin III should stop taking the pill?

Dr Winckelmann Antithrombin III levels, initially depressed by oral contraceptives tend to increase again during further courses of treatment. There is no reliable information about the coincidence of lowered antithrombin III levels and the occurrence of venous thrombosis. However, if antithrombin III levels are found repeatedly to be low in an individual before oral contraceptive usage then that woman should not use an oral contraceptive.

Question Do speakers feel that an antithrombin level test should be done on young girls before they start taking the pill?

Professor Briggs No, it costs $10 a test.

Dr Winckleman No. We cannot do this test as a routine test on all women.

Question Does Dr Winckelmann agree that continued pill usage is better than frequent pill 'pauses'?

Dr Winckleman With respect to hemostatic parameters – yes.

Question In view of the optimism about triphasic pills would they be appropriate for use in the postpartum period?

Professor Briggs Personally I feel a progestogen-only pill is the best in the immediate postpartum period – for 3 months – and then a combined-dose pill afterwards.

Section IV

Hypothalamic–Pituitary–Ovarian Axis and the Endometrium

Moderator: E. Diczfalusy

Chapter 12

Vaginal, cervical and endometrial changes during the triphasic pill

I. A. Brosens

The development of new types of oral contraceptive during the last decade was characterized by a progressive lowering of the estrogen component. At present much attention is given to the lowering of the progestogen component because of the possible role of the progestogen in the development of arterial disease and its effect on plasma lipoproteins and carbohydrates. However, the progressive reduction of both the estrogen and progestogen components resulted in an increased level of breakthrough bleeding and absence of withdrawal bleeding. To improve the cycle control a biphasic and two triphasic regimes of oral contraception have been tested[1]. These formulations tend to approximate the cyclic hormone pattern more closely to the normal than the fixed dose regimes. The most successful formulation is the triphasic pill composed of six tablets containing 30 μg ethinyl estradiol and 50 μg levonorgestrel, five tablets containing 40 μg ethinyl estradiol and 75 μg levonorgestrel and ten tablets containing 30 μg ethinyl estradiol and 125 μg levonorgestrel.

This paper reports on the work to investigate the effect of this triphasic pill on vaginal cytology, cervical mucus and the endometrium in order to evaluate the cyclic hormonal changes and the possible contraceptive effect at the uterine level.

VAGINAL CYTOLOGY AND CERVICAL MUCUS

The vaginal cytology and cervical mucus changes were studied every other day during the first cycle in 20 volunteers and after 1 year of treatment in 10 volunteers. Treatment in the first cycle was started on the first day of the cycle.

The karyopycnotic index reflecting the estrogenic effect in the vaginal cytology during the first cycle is shown in Figure 1. The karyopycnotic index calculated at 5–6 μ on smears stained by the Papanicolaou method was relatively high during the first phase, but decreased stepwise during the second phase to reach a low level during the third phase of the regime. The same pattern was seen in the group of volunteers after 1 year of treatment (Figure 2).

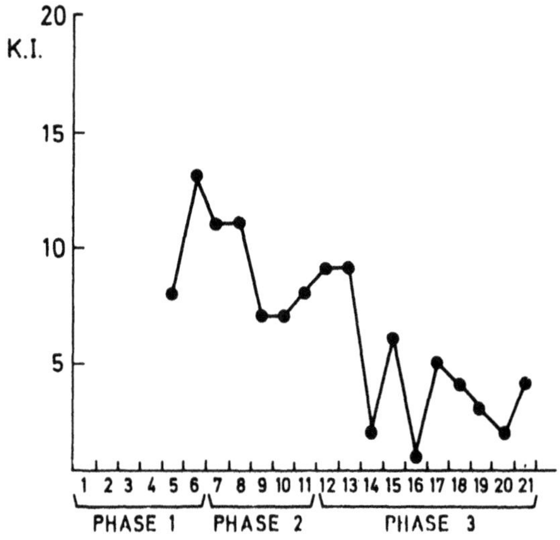

Figure 1 The karyopycnotic index of the vaginal epithelium during the first treatment cycle starting tablet 1 on day 1 of the cycle (from Brosens, I. *et al.* (1982). In Brosens, I. (ed.) *New Considerations on Oral Contraceptives*. (New York: BMI)

The cervical mucus changes were evaluated according to the scoring system of the WHO for quantity, Spinnbarkeit and

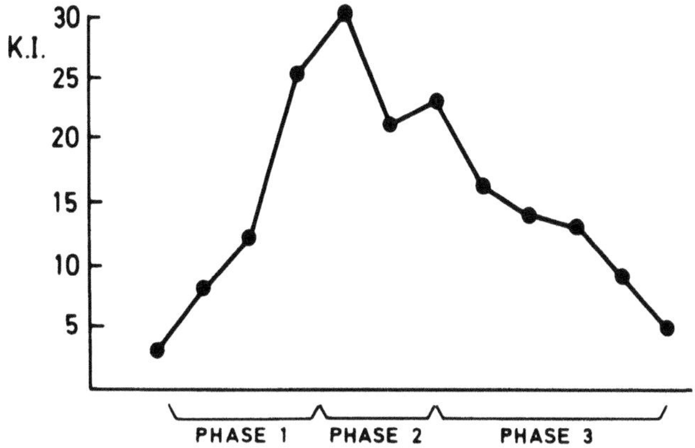

Figure 2 The karyopycnotic index of the vaginal epithelium after 1 year of treatment

ferning. During the first treatment cycle the quantity of mucus and the degree of Spinnbarkeit and ferning remained low in all patients throughout the cycle (Figure 3). After 1 year of treatment the same parameters were low indicating a progestogen-dominant effect on the cervical mucus throughout the cycle (Figure 4).

ENDOMETRIUM

With informed consent endometrial biopsies were obtained in 28 volunteers during the first cycle. Ten of these had not taken an oral contraceptive during the preceding three cycles and 18 were transferred from another norgestrel pill to the present preparation. In 14 patients biopsies were obtained between 8 and 16 months of treatment.

The biopsies were obtained at variable times during the cycle to obtain a composite picture of the endometrial changes. All

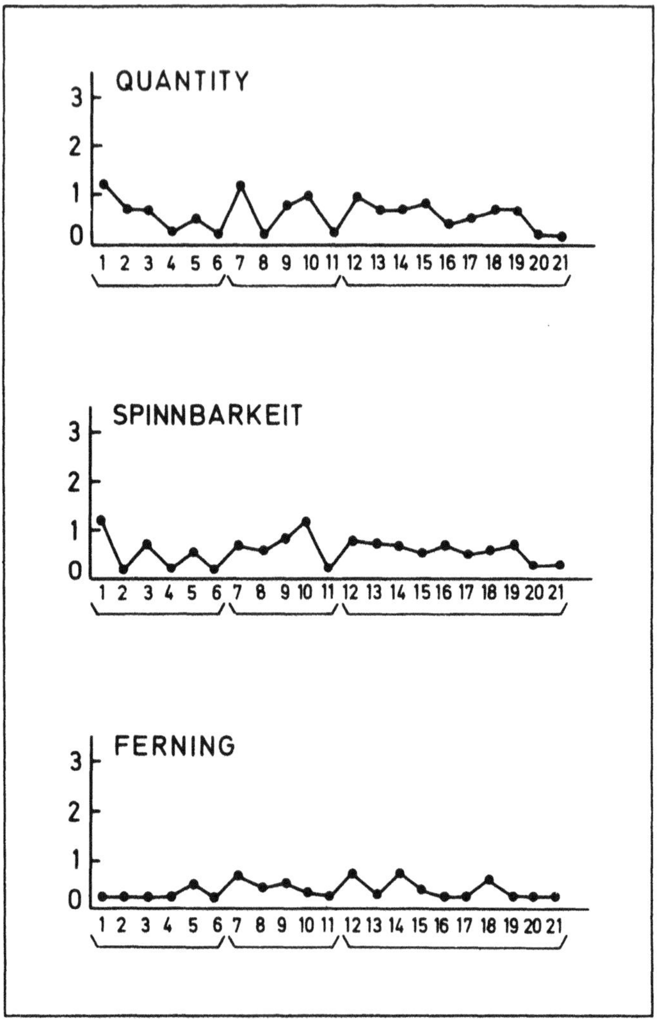

Figure 3 The cervical mucus changes during the first treatment cycle (from Brosens, I. *et al.* (1982). In Brosens, I. (ed.) *New Considerations on Oral Contraceptives.* (New York: BMI)

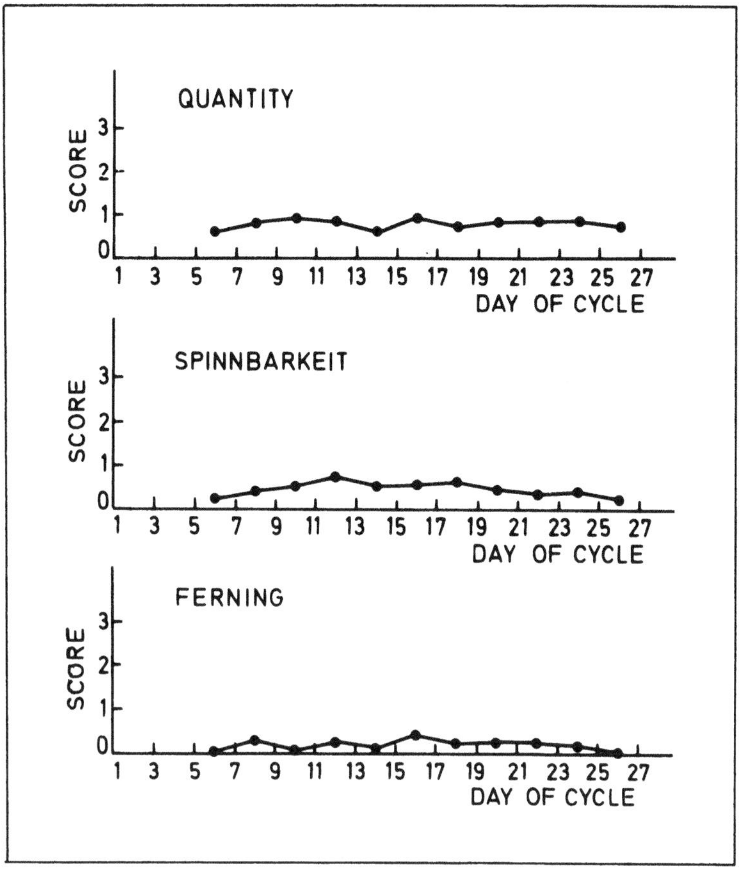

Figure 4 The cervical mucus changes after 1 year of treatment

specimens were assessed by the pathologist in the absence of the clinical data except for the knowledge that the biopsies were taken in patients under oral contraception. He was asked to date the endometrium according to the criteria of Noyes.

Although the endometria are different from normal, particularly by the dissociation of stromal and glandular changes, it was possible to observe cyclic changes in the endometria (Figure 5). During the first phase the endometrium changes from proliferation into early secretion. All biopsies during the second phase showed secretory changes although mitotic figures in the glandular epithelium were still frequently seen. At the end of this phase the endometrium compared with the endometrium on day 21–22 of the normal cycle. There was no significant increase of secretory changes during the third phase of treatment. At the end of the cycle the predecidual changes in the stroma are not reflected to the same extent as in the normal cycle and the maturation compared with the maturation day 23–24 of a normal cycle.

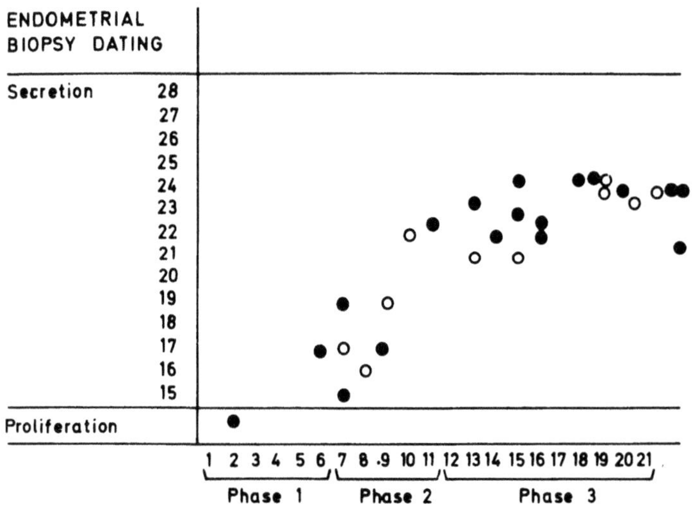

Figure 5 Correlation between the endometrial changes and the triphasic pill (from Brosens, I. *et al.* (1982). In Brosens, I. (ed.) *New Considerations on Oral Contraceptives*. (New York: BMI)

The inhibition of glandular growth and the early appearance of secretory activity in the triphasic preparation may explain the tendency to hypoplasia which is seen after prolonged use of the triphasic preparation. In comparing the triphasic preparation with a biphasic preparation (composed of 50 μg ethinyl estradiol with 50 μg levonorgestrel for 10 days followed by an increase of levonorgestrel to 125 μg during the last 11 days) the triphasic pill undoubtedly appears to be more progestogenic due to a short and weak estrogenic phase[2]. Stromal edema and sinusoid formation are seen in both regimes. An important feature of the biphasic and triphasic regimes is the better proliferation and development of the spiral arteries, in contrast with the poor development of these arteries during treatment with fixed regimes. This feature may explain, in part, why at this ultra-low dose level the triphasic formulation provides a better cycle control, particularly during the first cycles as compared with ultra-low fixed combinations[1].

The responses of the three target organs during triphasic pill administration are different. The vagina shows estrogenic impregnation during the first half of the cycle, very much the same as during a normal cycle. The cervical mucus is inhibited throughout the cycle and the endometrial biopsies reveal a short and weak estrogenic phase at the beginning of the cycle. The prolonged progestogenic phase is associated with hypoplastic changes in the endometrium.

It can therefore be concluded that the triphasic pill reflects the normal sequence of an estrogenic phase followed by a progestogenic phase but at the same time the effect on the cervical mucus and endometrium are unfavorable for conception. It is therefore no surprise that, combined with the inhibition of ovulation, the triphasic pill has the same contraceptive efficiency as the fixed dose pill.

ACKNOWLEDGEMENTS

The author is grateful to Professor Robertson and Dr P. Klerckx for evaluating the histological material, Dr Ide and Dr Debrock for assessing the cytology and Dr A. De Groote, Dr E. Bracke and Dr E. Bergin for evaluating the cervical mucus changes.

References

1. Lachnit-Fixson, U. (1980). Clinical investigation with a new triphasic oral contraceptive. In Greenblatt, R. B. (ed.) *Proceedings of a Symposium on a Triphasic Oral Contraceptive.* p. 99. (Lancaster: MTP Press)
2. Brosens, I. A., Robertson, W. B. and Van Assche, F. A. (1974). Assessment of incremental dosage regimen of combined oestrogen-progestagen oral contraceptive. *Br. Med. J.*, **4**, 643
3. Brosens, I., Klerckx, P., De Groote, A., Bracke, E., Bergin, E. and Van Assche, A. (1982). The hormonal effect of a triphasic oral contraceptive on the endometrium and cervical mucus. In Brosens, I. (ed.) *New Considerations on Oral Contraceptives.* (New York: BMI)

Chapter 13

Sensitivity changes of the pituitary during administration of a triphasic oral contraceptive

H.-D. Taubert, H. Fischer and J. S. E. Dericks-Tan

SUMMARY

The effect of a triphasic, low-dosed combined oral contraceptive (Triquilar[R]) upon pituitary capacity and sensitivity towards hypothalamic releasing-hormones was investigated on nine healthy women (ages 19–26 years) with normal ovulatory cycles. During a control cycle and during the first and third treatment cycle a stimulation test was carried out with 100 μg GnRH and 200 μg TRH on day 6, 11, 21 and 26. The typical cycle pattern of changing sensitivity of the pituitary gonadotroph toward stimulation with exogenous GnRH was clearly altered when the oral contraceptive was taken. When the first phase of the preparation (30 μg EE_2 and 50 μg levonorgestrel) had been taken for 6 days, there was a significant enhancement in the GnRH-induced release of LH as compared to the control cycle (early follicular phase). The LH-response towards GnRH was found to be decreased on the final days of the second phase (day 11) and third phase (day 21). On day 21, the reaction was significantly reduced as compared to the luteal phase of the control cycle. The TRH-induced release of PRL increased during treatment. Contrary to that, there was no noticeable effect of Triquilar upon basal and poststimulatory TSH values.

INTRODUCTION

Oral contraceptives are believed to act mainly by reducing the capacity of the pituitary gonadotrophs to release FSH and LH in response to stimulation by endogenous GnRH in a normal manner[1-4]. This hypothesis is primarily based on the observation that the release of both gonadotropins is greatly reduced when a challenge with exogenous GnRH is carried out in women using a combined oral contraceptive containing more than 50 μg of ethinyl estradiol (EE_2) per tablet at the end of a treatment cycle. As the suppression of the response to GnRH was clearly not as pronounced when a low-dosed oral contraceptive containing less than 50 μg of EE_2 was used, and there was no discernible inhibitory effect in women taking various minipill preparations[1], it had to be concluded that the mode of action of oral contraceptives upon the hypothalamo-pituitary axis was of a more complex nature than anticipated at first. This view was supported by the results of a study showing that the GnRH-stimulated release of LH actually increased within the first days of treatment of cyclic rats with 50 μg EE_2 and 1 mg norethisterone acetate, to be followed by a total suppression of the response when the treatment was continued for 30 days[5]. This unexpected type of reaction was presumed to be caused at least in part by the progestogen, a factor of time playing an important role, too. In view of these findings, we investigated pituitary responsiveness towards GnRH at the end of each phase of a triphasic combined low-dosed oral contraceptive (Triquilar^R) after 1, 3 and 6 months of use.

METHODS AND MATERIAL

Nine normally menstruating women (ages 19–26 years), whose intermenstrual interval ranged from 26 to 24 days, volunteered for participation in the study. None of them had used an oral contraceptive for at least 2 months prior to entering the study.

Each volunteer served as her own control. In the control cycle and during the first and third treatment cycle, a stimulation test was carried out with 100 μg GnRH (LH-RH-Relefact[R], Hoechst AG, Frankfurt am Main, FR Germany) and 200 μg TRH (TRH-Relefact[R], Hoechst AG, Frankfurt am Main, FR Germany) on day 6, 11, 21, and 26 after the onset of menstruation in the control cycle and after the onset of treatment with Triquilar, respectively. This triphasic oral contraceptive has the following composition:

Number of tablets	*Ethinyl estradiol* (μg)	*Levonorgestrel* (μg)
6	30	50
5	40	75
10	30	125

Immediately before and 20, 40, and 60 minutes after the i.v. injection of the releasing hormones, blood samples were taken from the antecubital vein for the determination of LH, FSH, PRL, and TSH by RIA.

Statistical calculations (arithmetical mean, SD, SE, unpaired *t*-test) were carried out on a desk computer. The pituitary capacity to respond to stimulation with releasing hormones was calculated by a trapezoid integration of the area under the curve per hour.

RESULTS

First treatment cycle

The release of LH in response to the injection of 100 μg GnRH at the end of the first phase of Triquilar (day 6) was significantly higher than in the early follicular phase (FP) of the control cycle ($p < 0.05$). The basal values were, however, not affected. After that, pituitary responsiveness decreased during the second and third phase of treatment. On day 21 of the first treatment cycle, both the basal (12.4 ± 7.3 *vs.* 4.3 ± 2.0 mIU/ml) and post-stimulatory (67.0 ± 24.7 *vs.* 23.0 ± 20.9 mIU/ml) LH level was significantly lower than in the control cycles ($p < 0.01$, Figure 1). Similarly, a significant inhibition of GnRH-stimulatable FSH release did not become apparent before day 21 of the first treatment cycle (Figure 2). The basal FSH level was lower than in the controls on day 6 and day 11 ($p < 0.05$).

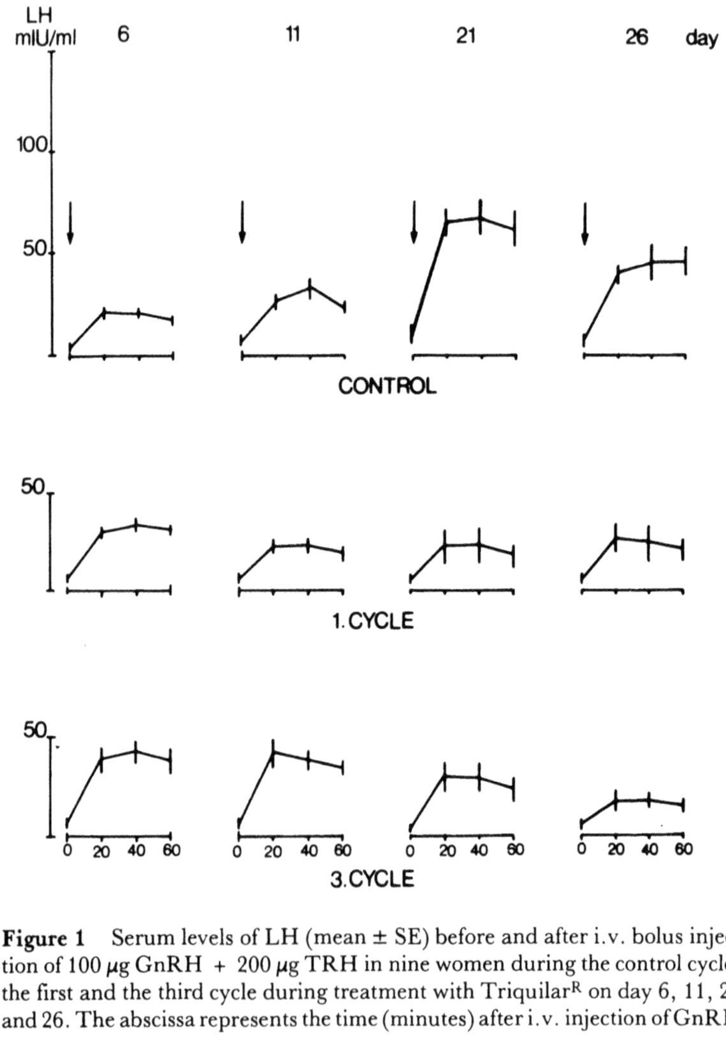

Figure 1 Serum levels of LH (mean ± SE) before and after i.v. bolus injection of 100 μg GnRH + 200 μg TRH in nine women during the control cycle, the first and the third cycle during treatment with Triquilar[R] on day 6, 11, 21 and 26. The abscissa represents the time (minutes) after i.v. injection of GnRH

The TRH-induced release of PRL was increased during all three phases of the first treatment cycle with Triquilar (Figure 3). Contrary to that, the release of TSH remained more or less unaffected (Figure 4). In both instances, there was no effect of the oral contraceptive on prestimulatory levels.

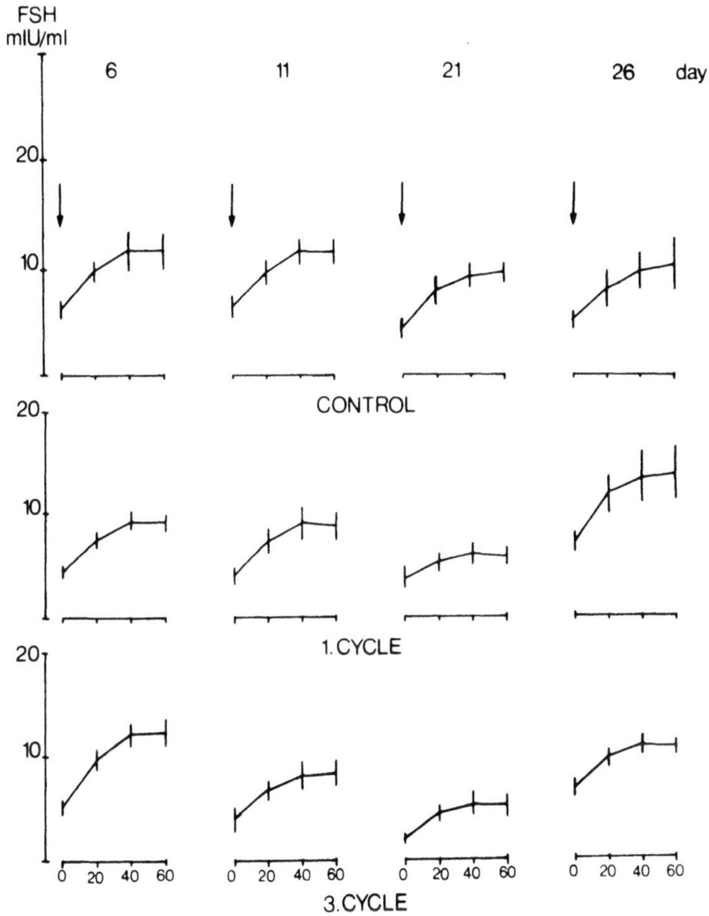

Figure 2 Serum levels of FSH (mean ± SE) before and after i.v. bolus injection of GnRH + TRH in women during the control cycle and during treatment with Triquilar[R] (see legend Figure 1)

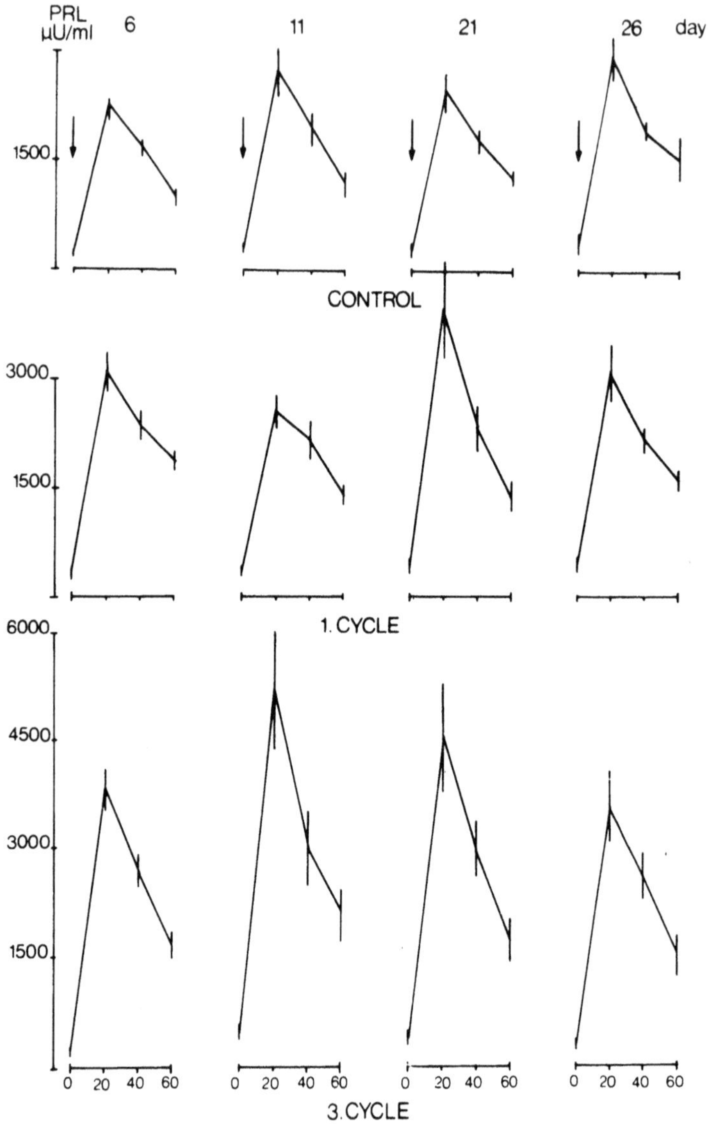

Figure 3 Serum levels of PRL (mean ± SE) before and after i.v. bolus injection of TRH in women before (control cycle) and during administration of Triquilar[R] (see legend Figure 1)

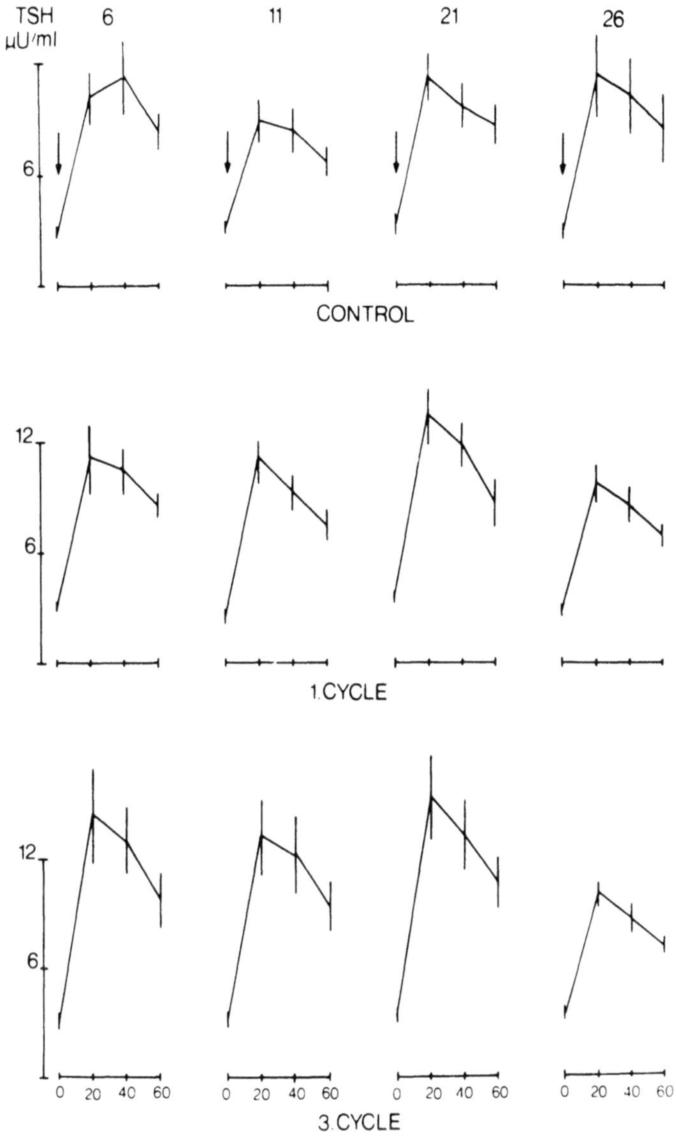

Figure 4 Serum levels of TSH (mean ± SE) before and after i.v. injection of TRH in women before (control cycle) and during administration of Triquilar[R] (see legend Figure 1)

Third treatment cycle

The changes in pituitary capacity and sensitivity observed towards GnRH during the first treatment cycle were found to be even more pronounced during the third month of treatment with Triquilar (Figures 1–4).

The poststimulatory levels of FSH were only suppressed on day 21, i.e. on the day the last tablet of the oral contraceptive was taken.

Similarly, basal LH levels were only suppressed on day 21 ($p < 0.01$) in both treatment cycle 1 and 3. As it had been shown in cycle 1, the response of LH to GnRH was enhanced to a highly significant degree on day 6, and, to a lesser degree, even on day 11. Thereafter, the GnRH-induced rise in serum LH was much smaller than in the luteal phase (LP) of the control cycles, even though a certain amount of LH continued to be released in an order of magnitude comparable to the FP.

The mean release of PRL and of LH per hour after stimulation with GnRH and TRH was also calculated as area under the curve before and during the use of the oral contraceptive (Figure 5). Six days after the initiation of treatment with Triquilar, the release of LH after administration of GnRH was in both the first and third treatment cycles significantly higher as compared to the control cycle ($p < 0.01$). After that, pituitary sensitivity decreased. On day 21 of the ingestion of Triquilar, the pituitary capacity to release LH was significantly lower than in the control cycle, a nadir being reached on day 26, i.e. during the 7-day pause between subsequent treatment cycles. It is quite remarkable, however, that there was not a single instance of complete suppression by Triquilar of pituitary capacity to respond to GnRH.

The TRH-induced release of PRL was even greater in treatment cycle 3 as compared to cycle 1.

When the tests were repeated after 6 months of treatment with Triquilar in two of the volunteers, the response pattern did not differ from that observed in treatment cycle 1 and 3.

It is noteworthy that a progesterone level of 1.8 ng/ml was found in the blood sample obtained prior to stimulation on day 21 of the first treatment cycle in one volunteer. Similarly, there were values in excess of 2 ng/ml on day 11 in two women during the third treatment cycle.

Intermenstrual bleeding

Six out of nine volunteers reported an intermenstrual spotting and bleeding lasting from 2 to 7 days during the first treatment cycle. The incidence and duration of these episodes decreased to three out of nine in treatment cycle 3.

DISCUSSION

The normal cyclic pattern of pituitary sensitivity towards GnRH underwent a pronounced change during the application of a low-dosed, combined oral contraceptive (Triquilar). In the normal, ovulatory cycle, the GnRH-stimulated release of LH is low in the follicular phase, reaches its highest values in the periovulatory phase, and attains an intermediate level during the luteal phase[6-8].

This does not become apparent in Figure 1, as no sampling was carried out during the periovulatory phase of the control cycles. It has already been shown by Kuhl *et al.*[5,9] that treatment of intact female rats with an ovulation-inhibiting dose of ethinyl estradiol and of a progestogen resulted at first in what appeared to be a paradoxical increase in pituitary sensitivity towards GnRH, which was, however, followed by a complete suppression of pituitary responsiveness. These findings were corroborated to a certain extent by the results of the present study in that the GnRH-induced release of LH was significantly higher on day 6 of treatment with Triquilar (first phase) as compared to the respective phase of the control cycle. This reaction was particularly noticeable during the third and sixth treatment cycles. There was no effect of the oral contraceptive on the prestimulatory level of LH. Subsequent to the initial enhancement of GnRH-stimulated LH release, there was a marked decline of pituitary responsiveness reaching a point of unequivocal suppression of both basal and poststimulatory LH levels. The degree of suppression did not differ between treatment cycle 1 and cycle 3.

Although the LH response to GnRH was lower on day 21 of treatment with the oral contraceptive than at the respective time of the control cycle, it was still comparable to the type of reaction seen in the early follicular phase of the ovulatory cycle. The most complete inhibition of pituitary function was seen on day 26, i.e. 5 days after the last tablet of the oral contraceptive had been taken.

The reaction of FSH release from the pituitary subsequent to stimulation with GnRH under the influence of an oral contraceptive differed from that of LH to a considerable degree. Contrary to LH, the response of FSH to GnRH was not enhanced during the application of the first phase of the triphasic oral contraceptive, i.e. of the tablets containing 30 μg of EE_2 and 50 μg of levonorgestrel. Moreover, there was no suppression of the response to GnRH on day 26 as it had been shown for LH. This shows clearly that there is a marked dichotomy with respect to the release of LH and FSH when the triphasic oral contraceptive is being used. Preliminary data indicate that this finding applies possibly to other types of oral contraceptive, too.

A previous study[10] had revealed that there is a certain reciprocal relationship between the suppression of GnRH-induced release of gonadotropins by oral contraceptives, and the enhancement of TRH-induced release of PRL. Even though the basal PRL levels did not differ from those of the control cycles, these observations were confirmed by the results of the present study, inasmuch as there was an unequivocal rise in PRL secretion after TRH injection when this was calculated by

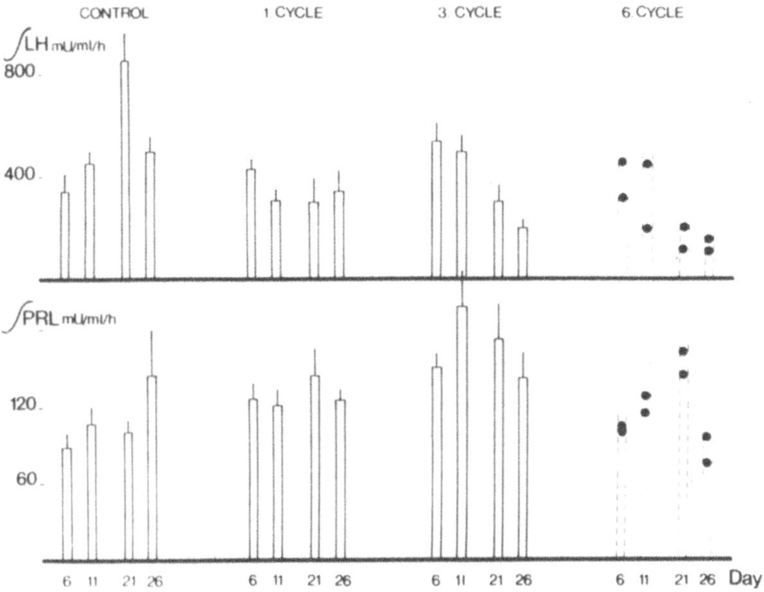

Figure 5 Pituitary responsiveness of LH and PRL (mean ± SE) after stimulation with GnRH + TRH as area under the curve during various days before (control cycle) and after treatment with Triquilar^R in the first and third cycles. The pituitary response of LH and PRL of two volunteers in a sixth treatment cycle is also depicted

determining the area under the curve (Figure 5). It is remarkable that the rise in TRH-stimulated PRL secretion was already demonstrable after 6 days of treatment with the first phase of the triphasic preparation containing the lowest dose of ethinyl estradiol and levonorgestrel, and there was practically no change when the measurements were repeated during the second and third phase of the oral contraceptive containing higher doses, and during later treatment cycles, too. Consequently, the differences in dosage between the three phases of Triquilar do not seem sufficient to effect a different response of the lactotrophs toward TRH. It is not known yet whether the stimulatory effect of oral contraceptive upon the lactotrophs is mediated via the hypothalamus, e.g. by decreasing the release of PIF, or is due to a direct effect of the sex steroids upon the pituitary. Contrary to that, the inhibition of gonadotropin release from the pituitary, or the shift in the ratio of LH and FSH brought about by oral contraceptive, is believed to be mainly caused by a direct suppression of GnRH secretion from the basal hypothalamus. The release of endogenous GnRH is presumed to follow the same type of pulsatile pattern of LH. In addition, there is ample evidence that this pulsatile release is subject to modulation by estrogens and progesterone with respect to frequency and amplitude[11,12]. The frequency of such pulses can be diminished by treatment with progestogens without affecting the height of the amplitude[13]. Conversely, estrogens seem to be capable of lowering the amplitude without changing the frequency. It is therefore quite conceivable that the relatively subtle changes in gonadotropin secretion brought about by the triphasic oral contraceptive in a time-dependent manner are mainly mediated by a change in the pulsatile pattern of GnRH release from the hypothalamus. Such interference with the normal cyclic pattern of LH and FSH release would certainly suffice to impair follicular development and prevent ovulation.

References

1. Dericks-Tan, J. S. E., Krög, W., Aktories, K. and Taubert, H.-D. (1976). Dose-dependent inhibition by oral contraceptives of the pituitary to release LH and FSH in response to stimulation with LH-RH. *Contraception*, **14**, 171
2. Scott, J. Z., Kletzky, O. A., Brenner, P. F. and Mishell, D. R. (1978). Comparison of the effects of contraceptive steroid formulations containing two doses of estrogen on pituitary function. *Fertil. Steril.*, **30**, 141
3. Rubinstein, L., Moguilevsky, J. and Leidenman, S. (1978). The effect of oral contraceptives on the gonadotropin response to LH-RH. *Obstet. Gynecol.*, **52**, 571
4. Wan, L. S., Weis, G. and Ganguly, M. (1978). Pituitary response to LH-RH stimulation in women on oral contraceptives. *Contraception*, **17**, 1

5. Kuhl, H., Sachs, A., Rosniatowski, C. and Taubert, H.-D. (1978). Time-dependent decrease of pituitary response to LH-RH after chronic treatment of intact female rats with ethinyloestradiol and norethindrone. *Acta Endocrinol. (Kbh.)*, **89**, 240
6. Yen, S. S. C., Vandenberg, G., Rebar, R. and Ehara, Y. (1972). Variation in pituitary responsiveness to synthetic LRF during different phases of the menstrual cycle. *J. Clin. Endocrinol. Metab.*, **35**, 931
7. Nillius, S. J. and Wide, L. (1972). Variation in LH and FSH response to LH-releasing hormone during the menstrual cycle. *J. Obstet. Gynecol. Br. Commonw.*, **79**, 865
8. Thomas, K., Cardon, M., Donnez, J. and Ferin, J. (1973). Changes in hypophyseal responsiveness to synthetic LH-RH during the normal menstrual cycle in women. *Contraception*, **7**, 289
9. Kuhl, H., Baziad, A. and Taubert, H.-D. (1982). Augmentative and inhibitory effects of chronic steroid injections on LH release in dependency on time. *Endocrinol. Exp.* (In press)
10. Dericks-Tan, J. S. E., Eberlein, L., Streb, C. and Taubert, H.-D. (1977). The effect of oral contraceptives and of bromocriptine upon pituitary stimulation by LH-RH and TRH. *Contraception*, **17**, 79
11. Yen, S. S. C., Tsai, C. C., Naftolin, F., Vandenberg, G. and Ajabor, L. (1972). Pulsatile patterns of gonadotropin release in subjects with and without ovarian function. *J. Clin. Endocrinol. Metab.*, **34**, 671
12. Santen, R. J. and Bardin, C. W. (1973). Episodic luteinizing hormone secretion in man. Pulse analysis, clinical interpretation, physiological mechanisms. *J. Clin. Invest.*, **52**, 2617
13. Goodman, R. L. and Karsch, F. J. (1980). Pulsatile secretion of luteinizing hormone: differential suppression by ovarian steroids. *Endocrinology*, **107**, 1286

Chapter 14

Influence of hormonal contraception on the maturation process of the hypothalamo–pituitary–ovarian axis

R. H. Wyss, I. Rey-Stocker, M.-M. Zufferey and M.-T. Lemarchand

We know that the onset of menarche has been occurring progressively earlier over the last decades. For example, in Norway, from 1840 to 1950, the average age of menarche fell from 17 to 13½ years of age (Figure 1). This trend has been observed in all developed countries. Precocious menarche may

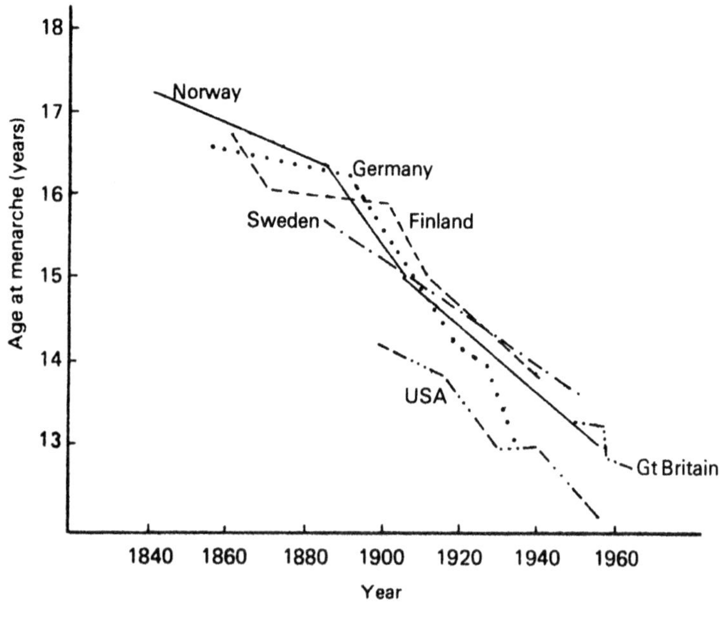

Figure 1 Change of age-at-onset of menarche with time

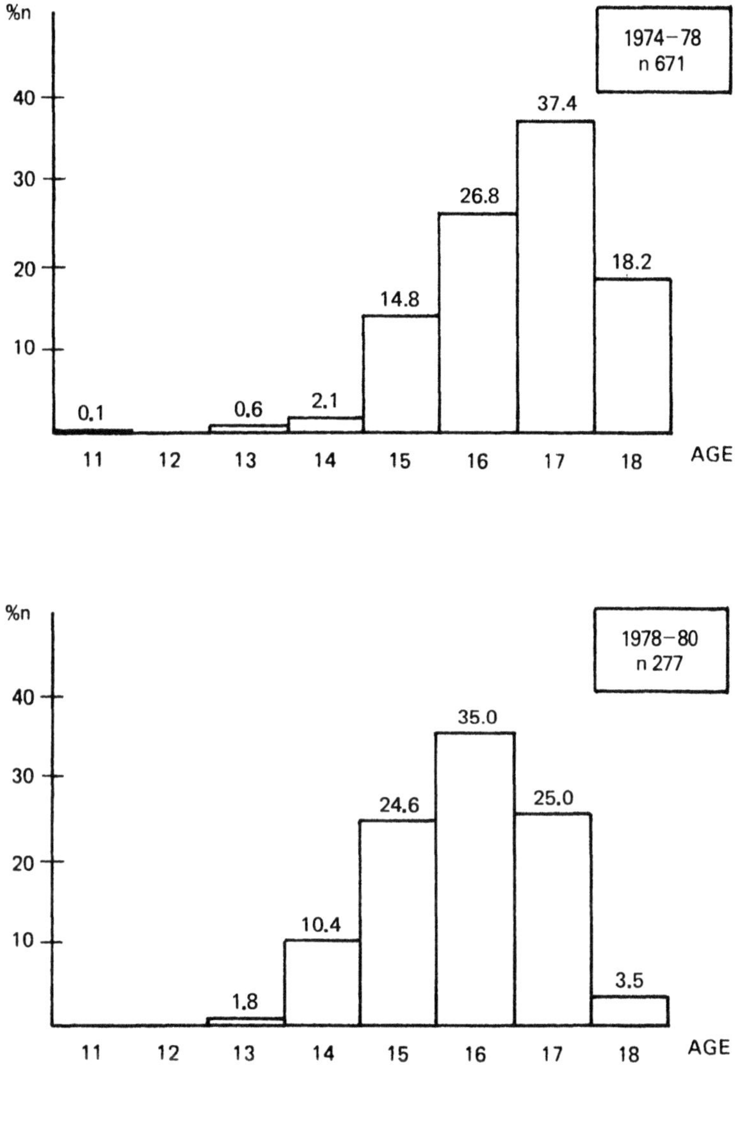

Figure 2 Age at the time of first gynecological consultation

lead to precocious maturation of secondary sexual organs, which in turn may explain precocious sexuality. In Geneva, for instance, increasingly younger adolescents have been asking for contraception, and their average age has dropped from 16.5 to 15.9 years of age, over the last 2–3 years (Figure 2).

Hypothalamic and pituitary function of adolescents up to 5 years after menarche rarely reaches the functional capacity of the adult woman. For this reason, the first menstrual cycles are very often irregular. Ovulation does not occur systematically with menarche, and 1 year after the onset of menarche, only

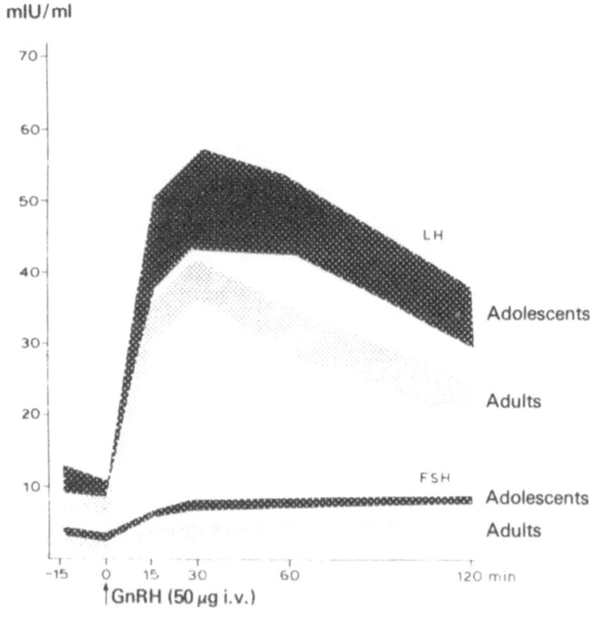

Figure 3 LH and FSH responses to GnRH in young adults and in adolescents 5 years after menarche – luteal phase. Reproduced from Rey-Stocker, I. (1980). In Huber, A. (ed.) *Probleme der Kontrazeption bei der Jugendlichen*. by permission of Excerpta Medica.

14% of cycles are ovulatory. Even 6 years after the onset of menarche, only 86% of the cycles are ovulatory, as shown by Widholm. Even when ovulation does occur, the following luteal phase is often inadequate.

There was a difference in reaction after stimulation by 50 μg GnRH, between 17 girls, 5 years after menarche, and 23 adult women of average age 27, who had never delivered and whose cycles were ovulatory (Figure 3). The basal values were not much different, but after stimulation both LH and FSH responded more actively in the young girls. The same can be found for thyreotropin after stimulation with 200 μg of TRF. There is a significantly stronger release of thyreotropin in the young girls than in the adult women (Figure 4). The secretion of

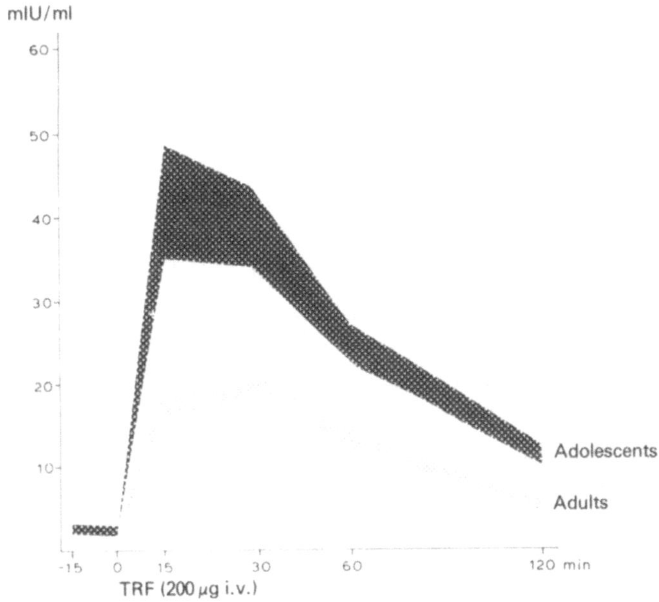

Figure 4 TSH responses to TRF in young adults and in adolescents 5 years after menarche – luteal phase. Reproduced from Rey-Stocker, I. (1980). In Huber, A. (ed.) *Probleme der Kontrazeption bei der Jugendlichen.* by permission of Excerpta Medica.

prolactin is identical in both groups. Comparing the level of estrogen and progesterone shows a significant increase in both hormones from the age of menarche to adult age. Following a constant increase, estradiol reaches the level of the adult women 2–3 years after the onset of menarche, whereas progesterone, following a constant rise, does not reach the level of adult women even 5 years after menarche (Table 1).

We know that combination oral contraceptives inhibit the basal secretion of gonadotrophins and their reaction to GnRH. They also inhibit the basal secretion of TSH and its response to TRF. They do not inhibit secretion of prolactin in the adult woman. But how do they react on the young girl? Is the endocrine maturation process influenced by hormonal contraception? To answer this question, 103 young girls who had been on hormonal contraception for up to 24 months, within the 5 years following the onset of menarche, were examined and compared to 17 girls who had never used hormonal contraception, during the same period of 5 years following menarche.

After stopping oral contraception, values of gonadotropins, prolactin and TSH were measured from day 21 to 25 of the following cycle, before and after simultaneous stimulation by i.v. injection of 50 μg LHRH and 200 μg of TRF. Estradiol and progesterone were also measured at the same time (Table 1). The values were compared with those of the control group. Two

Table 1 The level of estradiol and progesterone in the second half of the cycle

Years after menarche	*Estradiol* (pg/ml)	*Progesterone* (ng/ml)	*Ovulatory cycles in %* (progesterone > 2 ng/ml)
1 year (n=4)	35 ± 5*	0.61 ± 0.17*	0
2 years (n=9)	90 ± 25	2.93 ± 1.23*	38
3 years (n=23)	105 ± 15	5.85 ± 1.38*	56
4 years (n=27)	120 ± 30	5.10 ± 1.35*	56
5 years (n=16)	115 ± 15	5.93 ± 1.25*	63
10 years (n=23)	105 ± 10	11.20 ± 1.52	100

* $P < 0.05$

different combination pills were used, the first one containing 50 μg of ethinyl estradiol and 1 mg of lynestrenol (Ovostat[R] or Ovoresta[R]).

Following 3, 6 and 12 months with this pill the basal values of LH and FSH were identical to those of the control group (Figure 5). The reaction of LH to GnRH stimulation increased with the length of pill use, and after 12 months use was significantly

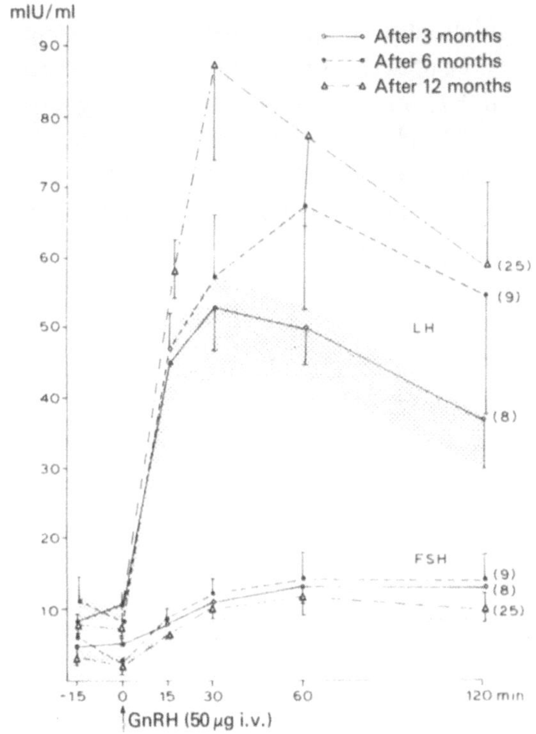

Figure 5 LH and FSH responses to GnRH after oral contraception (Ovostat[R]) in adolescents – luteal phase. Reproduced from Rey-Stocker, I. (1980). In Huber, A. (ed.) *Probleme der Kontrazeption bei der Jugendlichen.* by permission of Excerpta Medica.

different from the values of the control group. The values of FSH after stimulation were increased following 3 and 6 months of pill use, but the difference with the control group was not significant. After 12 months of pill use, the reaction of FSH was identical to that of the control group. The reaction of TSH to TRF after 3 months was more important than that of the control group but the difference was not significant. After 6 and 12 months use it approached that of the control group. The reaction of prolactin to TRF increased and became significantly higher after 12 months of use, compared to the control group (Figure 6). The second type of oral contraceptive contained 30 μg of ethinyl estradiol and 0.15 mg of levonorgestrel (Microgynon[R] 30). The basal values of FSH decreased significantly after 3–18 months use with this combination pill. The basal values of LH and the reaction of FSH and LH to GnRH stimulation did not differ significantly from those of the control group (Figure 7). The basal values of TSH and prolactin were identical to those of the

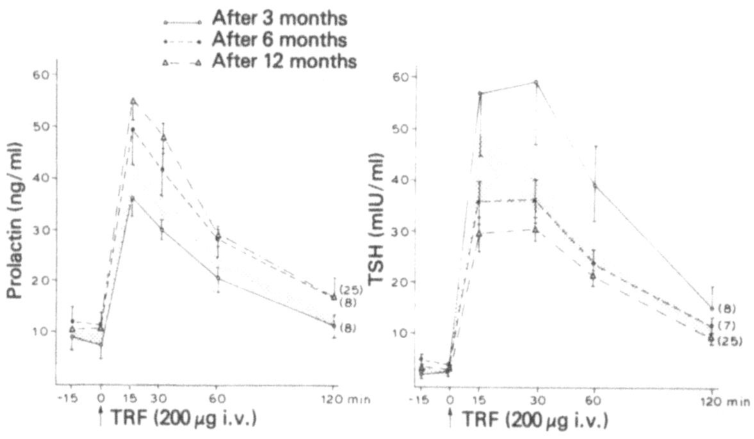

Figure 6 PRL and TSH responses to TRF after oral contraception (Ovostat[R]) in adolescents – luteal phase. Reproduced from Rey-Stocker, I. (1980). In Huber, A. (ed.) *Probleme der Kontrazeption bei der Jugendlichen*. by permission of Excerpta Medica.

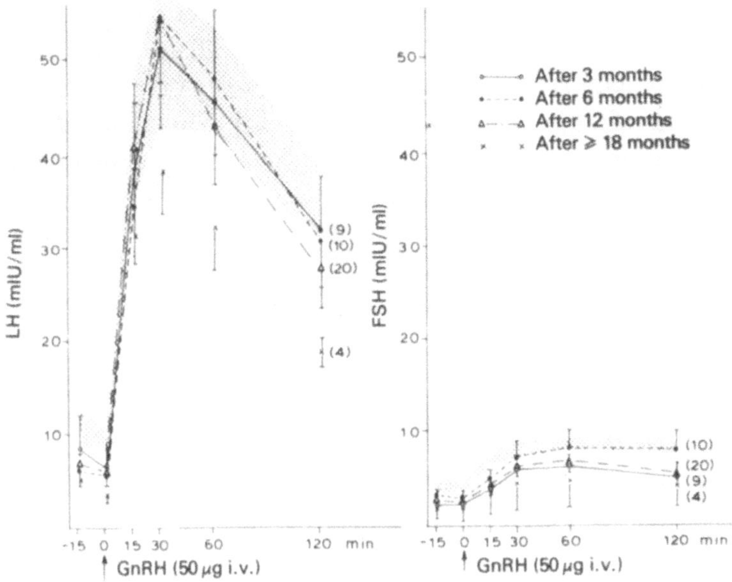

Figure 7 LH and FSH responses to GnRH after oral contraception (Microgynon[R]30) in adolescents – luteal phase. Reproduced from Rey-Stocker, I. (1980). In Huber, A. (ed.) *Probleme der Kontrazeption bei der Jugendlichen.* by permission of Excerpta Medica.

control group (Figure 8). The reaction of TSH to TRF, after 3 months on the pill, was significantly lower. But with time the reaction increased and corresponded, at 6 months and more, to that of the control group.

The reaction of prolactin on stimulation of TRF increased and was significantly higher after 12 and 18 months. To verify ovulation after cessation of oral contraception, one or more measures of progesterone were made between day 21 and 25 of the first postpill menstrual cycle (Table 2). With Ovostat ovulation in the first postpill cycle occurred in 46% of girls after 3 months of pill use, 40% after 6 months, and 50% after 12 months of pill use. With Microgynon 30, ovulation occurred in the first postpill cycle in 66% after 3 months of pill use, 60% after 6 months, and 75% after 12 months of pill use. In another series studying ovulation following cessation of oral contraception after 24 months of use with various other preparations, 67% ovulated in the first postpill cycle. In the control group 63% ovulated (Table 2). The lower percentage of 40–50% ovulations with Ovostat could be attributed to the fact that only one blood measure of progesterone was made in the secondary phase of the cycle, as compared with several ones in the other groups. The

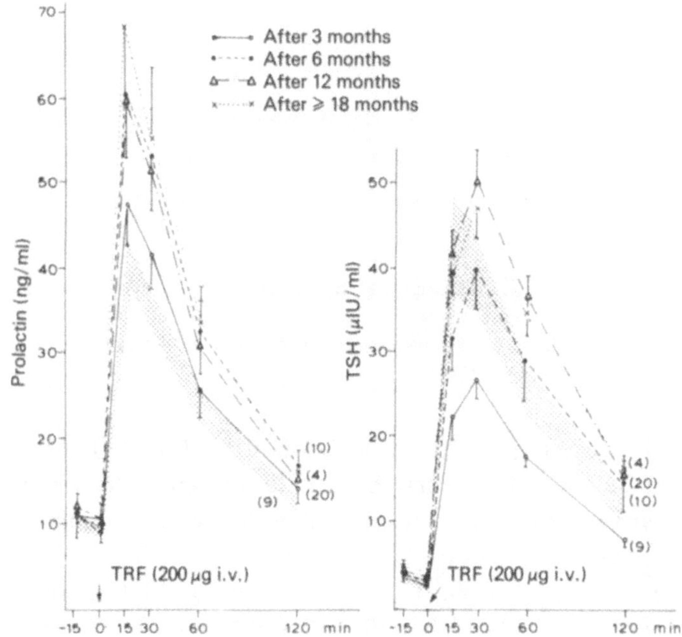

Figure 8 Prolactin and TSH responses to TRF after oral contraception (Microgynon^{R}30) in adolescents – luteal phase. Reproduced from Rey-Stocker, I. (1980). In Huber, A. (ed.) *Probleme der Kontrazeption bei der Jugendlichen.* by permission of Excerpta Medica.

values of LH and FSH before and after stimulation with GnRH and those of prolactin and TSH before and after stimulation with TRF were not statistically different from that of the control group even after 24 months of different pill use (Figures 9 and 10).

Regardless of the different oral contraceptive preparations and independently of the duration of use, the results of the investigations show that the activity of the pituitary gland returns to its normal function immediately after stopping contraception.

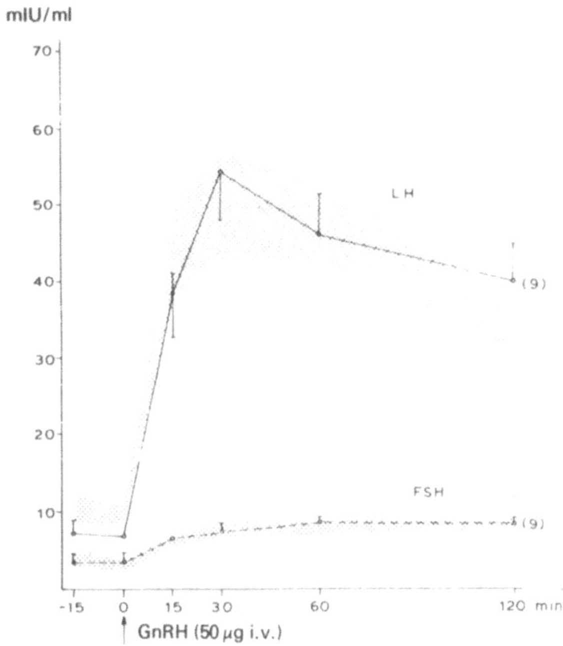

Figure 9 LH and FSH responses to GnRH after > 2 years of oral contraception in adolescents – luteal phase. Reproduced from Rey-Stocker, I. (1980). In Huber, A. (ed.) *Probleme der Kontrazeption bei der Jugendlichen.* by permission of Excerpta Medica.

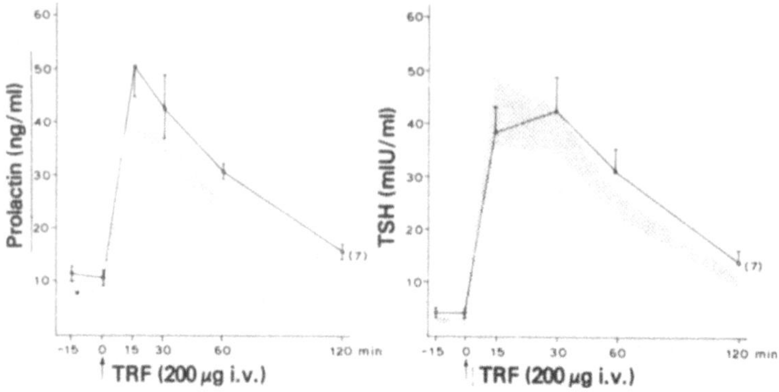

Figure 10 PRL and TSH responses to TRF after > 2 years of oral contraception in adolescents – luteal phase. Reproduced from Rey-Stocker, I. (1980). In Huber, A. (ed.) *Probleme der Kontrazeption bei der Jugendlichen.* by permission of Excerpta Medica.

Table 2 Level of estradiol and progesterone in the following second half of the cycle after stopping oral contraception

Oral contraception Length of intake	*Estradiol* (pg/ml)	*Progesterone* (ng/ml)	*Ovulatory cycles in* % (progesterone > 2 ng/ml)
1 mg lynestrenol + 0.05 mg EE			
After 3 months	110.0 ± 22.8 (n=8)	4.0 ± 1.4 (n=13)	46.1
After 6 months	113.6 ± 45.2 (n=7)	3.6 ± 1.7 (n=10)	40
After 12 months	134.5 ± 21.2 (n=21)	3.7 ± 1.1 (n=23)	50
0.15 mg levonorgestrel + 0.03 mg EE			
After 3 months	81 ± 11 (n=5)	5.4 ± 1.7 (n=9)	66
After 6 months	123 ± 11 (n=10)	5.9 ± 1.7 (n=10)	60
After 12 months	154 ± 12 (n=19)	7.8 ± 1.3 (n=20)	75
Various oral contraceptions after more than 24 months	97.7 ± 22.8 (n=9)	8.4 ± 1.9 (n=18)	67
Control group adolescents 5–6 years after menarche without hormonal contraception	115 ± 15 (n=16)	5.9 ± 1.3 (n=16)	63

The reinforced LH release, after taking Ovostat over a 12 month period, seems to produce a rebound effect. The continuous intake of Microgynon 30 already induces a latent hyperprolactinemia after a 6 month period and Ovoresta induces a latent hyperprolactinemia after 12 months only, as measured after stimulation with TRF. Such a result in the group of girls on oral contraception for more than 2 years could no longer be found. It therefore appears to be a temporary reaction which disappears after prolonged use of oral contraception.

The measurement of the sexual steroids in the second half of the cycle shows that the ovaries immediately regain their activity after stopping oral contraception.

The average level of estradiol and progesterone, as well as the frequency of ovulation, correspond to those of a control group of young girls, 5–6 years after the onset of menarche and not taking hormones.

The results of these investigations demonstrate the extraordinary adaptability of the pituitary gland in young girls and lead to the assumption that oral contraception does not alter the maturation of the endocrine system.

Bibliography

Rey-Stocker, I., Zufferey, M.-M., Lemarchand, M.-T. and Rais, M. Sensibilität der Hypophyse, der Gonaden und der Schilddrüse beim jungen Mädchen vor und nach kombinierter oraler Kontrazeption.

Zufferey, M.-M. Maturation de l'axe hypothalamo-hypophysaire de l'ovaire et de la thyroïde au cours de l'adolescence et effet de la contraception hormonale.

Thesis, University of Lausanne, Faculty of Médecine

Discussion

Question What is the mechanism of action of a steroid contraceptive? Is it mediated via the hypothalmic axis, or another mechanism or ovulatory inhibition?

Dr Taubert The favored reaction is that the low-dose oral contraceptive disrupts the pulsatile release – as described in the paper given. The biochemical evidence is confusing and I would not propose any other mode of action. It is certainly not the inhibition of gonodatrophin release alone.

Question How do you view the mechanism of action of a steroid contraceptive when it inhibits ovulation? Is it mediated entirely via the hypothalamo-pituitary system or can you see other mechanisms as well?

Dr Taubert At present I would favor the notion that at least low-dose oral contraceptives act by disrupting the pulsatile release as I said in my last few sentences. That of course is an unproven hypothesis; we are working at it but I would not even dare to claim that it was proven. As far as the action at a pituitary level is concerned, I think the biochemical evidence is so confusing, at least from the view of our laboratory, that I would not dare propose any mode of action. Certainly it cannot be understood as a phenomenon of disturbing gonodatrophin release, since a whole sequence of interactions are involved in the inhibition of ovulation.

Professor Diczfalusy As a matter of fact we have published a number of papers which showed that there was no correlation between pituitary gonodatrophin inhibition and the other indices of ovulatory cycles such as daily levels of progesterone or estradiol.

Round Table

Moderator: *J. Hammerstein*

Panel of Speakers: *M. Breckwoldt*
E. Diczfalusy
A. A. Haspels
K. Irsigler
R. Rolland
R. Wiseman

Dr Hammerstein The issue we have to deal with at this Round Table is 'has the attitude changed with regard to the risks and benefits of oral contraception?' This is a rather rhetorical question since, I am sure, nobody in the hall would dare to answer 'no'. Let us therefore consider during the next two hours in which respect and not whether our attitudes towards oral contraception have changed during the last two decades.

On the introduction of oral contraception in the early 1960s the main emphasis was on contraceptive safety. Next to this the endocrine effects of long duration usage was paid attention to, whereas metabolic effects were rather neglected. The latter since it was felt improbable at that time that synthetic hormones could act in any different way to endogenous hormones. Thus thinking predominently in terms of contraceptive safety, this has been the decisive factor which lead to the much too high dosages of the first oral contraceptives. Not before the seventies did the amounts of steroids in the pill come down. The first norethisterone-containing tablet available, for instance, contained 10 mg of this progestogen per pill whilst presently there are formulations with only 1/20th of this amount on the market. As another example, Enovid contained 150 μg mestranol per pill which is up to seven times the amount of estrogen that is nowadays in the so called 'micro-pills' (estrogen content < 50 μg). The decrease in the dosage of estrogen started in 1970 according to a recommendation from the British Committee of Safety of Drugs after a combined English and Scandinavian study had shown that there was apparently a correlation between thromboembolic disease on the one hand, and the dosage of estrogen in the oral contraceptives used on the other.

In Germany now the three leading companies in this field find that 28–44% of all pills used are 'micro-pills'. In The Netherlands this proportion is presently over 50% of all pills used. This was also the situation in the UK in 1979 and last year the sales rate of the low-dose 'micro-pills' increased to more than ⅔rds of all oral contraceptives sold. This trend varies from country to country and I would like to know whether additional information or remarks can be given at the Round Table on this matter.

Dr Diczfalusy Perhaps credit should be given to the Chinese investigators for the trend towards low-dose pills. Before the first low-dose pill was launched in the United States or in Europe the National Co-ordinating Group of China developed a pill which, as you may recall, was derived from a norethisterone/ethinyl estradiol original combination. Finally they settled for 625 μg norethisterone and 35 μg of ethinyl estradiol formulation. There was a national co-ordinating group which was in charge of this in Shanghai (Yang Tsao-Chen: In Briggs, M. H. and Diczfalusy, E. (eds.) Pharmacological models in contraceptive development. *Acta Endocrinol.* (Kbh.) Suppl. 185 (1974) 166–7).

Dr Hammerstein Don't we all believe that the newer 'micro-pills' have less risk to the patient than the older pills with 50 μg of estrogen or more in it? There are, however, only two papers one from England and the other from Sweden which I am aware of, which demonstrate that there actually appeared to be a decrease in the frequency of side-effects concomitantly with the decrease in the estrogen dosage of the pill. Is there anybody aware of additional proofs for superiority of the 'micro-pill' regarding the risks?

Dr Wiseman I showed earlier that there has been no decrease which can be attributed to oral contraceptives in ischaemic heart disease, and this applies to all aspects of circulatory disease. The advent of low-dose pills has not seemingly changed the pattern of mortality statistics in the United Kingdom in women of reproductive age, and the data that I presented this morning is borne out by data from other parts of the world. The group in Sweden, (Vertigo *et al.*) has shown that the rate of arterial disease in women of reproductive age between 1966 and 1970, when there were only 50 μg pills or higher dosage available, is identical to that of between 1976 and 1979 when the overwhelming usage was of 30 μg pills. Similarly, I quoted this morning the work of the Oxford Group, (Adam and Thorogood last year in the *British Journal of Family Planning*) and they showed that there was no difference in relative risk between women who were using 50 μg pills and those who were using 30 μg pills. The available evidence suggests that there is no difference in risk, and I would go further and say that there doesn't appear to be any risk at all from oral contraceptives of arterial disease.

Dr Hammerstein You speak about arterial disease and others have talked about venous thromboembolism. I think one should strictly distinguish between the two. There is convincing data indicating that the estrogens raise the frequency of venous thromboembolism, whereas the progestogens are positively related to arterial diseases, the cardioischemic diseases and hypertension especially. One has therefore to make the distinction between these two. Böttiger *et al.* (1980), the Swedish group already mentioned, remarked that the morbidity of venous thromboembolism went down markedly in 1975/1976 when the micro-pill became very popular in Sweden whereas the arterial complications did not change at all.

Dr Breckwoldt I think that we should keep in mind that these are all preliminary data and the time-span is too short to draw any definite conclusions. What do we expect from the ideal hormonal contraceptive in general? Reliable ovulation suppression; acceptable regulation of the menstrual pattern; full reversibility; minimal, none at all, or even beneficial side-effects; and a reasonable price! When discussing side-effects of the pill we should not forget that there are a number of beneficial side-effects which can be used in a therapeutic manner. Improvement of virilizing symptoms such as acne, hirsutism and seborrhea, for example, and the relief of dysmenorrhea. This morning some speakers mentioned that the rate of dysmenorrhea is decreasing with the use of oral contraceptives. This may have something to do with the production of prostaglandins by the endometrium which is brought under control by the sex steroids.

Dr Hammerstein Coming back to the micro-pill, it is obviously not quite so 'safe' as the pill with 50 μg of estrogen. It may be recalled that when Pincus, Garcia and Rock made their first investigations in Puerto Rico they found that with the first high dosage formulations (see Table 1) as many as five pills per cycle could be omitted without any decrease in contraceptive safety. One surely cannot do the same with the micro-preparation nowadays, but we have got no relevant data as yet. There are, however, studies on this subject supported by WHO underway.

Table 1 Oral contraceptives: decrease in dosage during the course of time

Trade name	μg	*Estrogen*	mg	*Progestogen*	*Country*	*Year of introduction*
Enovid	150	EEME	10	NDL	USA	1960
Ortho Novum	60	"	10	NET	USA	1960
Anovlar	50	EE	4	NETA	BRD	1961
Ovysmen	35	"	0.5	NET	BRD	1975
Loestrin	20	EE	1.0	NETA	USA	vor 1976

EEMA = Mestranol
EE = Ethinyl estradiol
NDL = Norethynodrel
NET = Norethisterone
NETA = Norethisterone acetate

Dr Diczfalusy The Task Force on Oral Contraceptives was much concerned about the problem of patient compliance. In different cultural settings, in different countries what is compliance when it comes to daily pill taking? My group was asked to conduct a controlled study (similar to the ones published by Morris *et al.*, *Contraception,* **20** (1979) 61–9 and Chowdhury *et al.*, *Contraception*, **22** (1980) 241–7). It included a group of 32 women, 8 in each group, and they were deliberately asked to omit the pill over 48 hour periods. One group omitted days 9 and 10, the next omitted days 11 and 12, the third days 14 and

15 and the last days 18 and 19. Daily assays of estradiol and progesterone levels were carried out. Those assays indicated that there were different types of ovarian reaction in terms of estradiol levels, but that 31 of the 32 subjects had no elevation whatsoever in their progesterone levels. The reason for this is that the half-life of levonorgestrel is quite long; in 31 of the 32 subjects it averaged 29 hours (Wang *et al.*, in preparation). In one subject a normal ovulatory-like progesterone profile was found. Analysis of the levonorgestrel levels revealed that this subject did not take any pills during the last cycle and did not start pill-taking before day 9 of the study cycle. Thus if one pill is missed, or even if two pills are missed, this will not influence the circulating level of levonorgestrel levels to such an extent that one should be alarmed.

What happens if a woman omits this pill in subsequent cycles? What happens if she omits the pill on days, say 8–9, in three consecutive cycles? Does this mean that there is a growth of a new set of follicles? In order to ascertain this we are conducting another study. The results are currently being analysed and so far in all subjects except one, we have found no evidence of a 'rebound effect' in terms of an increased estradiol or progesterone level. In one subject, in two out of three cycles, we have found ovulatory progesterone levels, however, and it seems that she ovulated within 10 days after discontinuation of the pill. Although, obviously a great deal more information is needed, these data seem to suggest a certain hazard associated with pill omission if it prolongs the pill-free period.

Dr Hammerstein These are very useful investigations. Dr Diczfalusy will surely agree however that, in practice, other factors add to the problem – malabsorption for instance, or an enzyme alteration which decreases the bioavailability of the contraceptive steroid. Do not such influences decrease the reliability in the contraceptive effect of the micro-pill more than just omitting the pill for one or two days?

Dr Diczfalusy Agreed it can also be in the SHBG levels which we have not yet discussed but which may be very important.

Dr Hammerstein The next point of practical importance which needs clarification is 'how to behave in the case of spotting or breakthrough bleeding?' Is it worthwhile just increasing the estrogen dosage, or asking the patient to take two instead of one tablet for a few days?

Dr Haspels The principle is, that when you get breakthrough bleeding or spotting in the first half of the pill intake, you add some estrogen. In China they have a pill Number 3, which contains 50 μg of ethinyl estradiol which we do not have here. If you have bleeding in the second half of the pill intake you switch from pill Number 1 to pill Number 2 so you double the progestogen content. What I prescribe when there is breakthrough bleeding and spotting, is 3 months of higher-dosage pill. This usually corrects it all, and then I return the patient to the low-dose oral contraceptive.

Dr Breckwoldt It depends on the extent of the breakthrough bleeding and whether the patient is bothered about this side-effect or not. In most cases I advise the patient just to continue taking the pill and the breakthrough bleeding will disappear anyway.

Dr Hammerstein The medical advice should also depend on when the breakthrough bleeding does occur. If it is at the beginning, i.e. during the first three treatment cycles, then one sometimes really has to switch to another preparation because the original pill is not well tolerated. If it happens at a later time then there is a suspicion of a decreased bioavailability of the contraceptive steroid or that the patient is no longer taking the pill in the proper way. One has to clarify this with the patient and then to inform a patient how to behave in the future. The failure of the patient to take her pills properly is one of the main reasons for breakthrough bleeding, I think, and it sometimes takes quite a while to find this out from the patient and to adapt the contraceptive procedure accordingly.

Dr Haspels There is a study in Holland at the Sexology Institute which indicates that 20% of Dutch women forget at least two or more pills every month. This is really quite remarkable.

Dr Diczfalusy In 1979 the World Health Organization arranged a Symposium on 'Endometrial Bleeding and Steroidal Contraception' (Diczfalusy, E., Fraser, I. S. and Webb, F. T. G. (eds.) (Bath: Pitman Press). The conclusion of that symposium was that nobody, among us at least, understands intermenstrual bleeding. What is the pathogenesis of why women bleed, when women bleed and how? After this symposium one study where the norethisterone 'mini-pill' 30 μg was given to women, and when they started bleeding within 6 hours they were allocated, at random, either to a placebo or to an ethinyl estradiol treatment. They either got 50 μg ethinyl estradiol for 7 days or a placebo and a number of endometrial parameters were measured. There was no difference between those two small groups (Johannisson *et al.* (1982), *Contraception,* **25**, 13–30). I don't want to say that estrogen is of no use, all I would emphasise is that we must learn more about the pathogenesis of intermenstrual bleeding if we want to develop a rational therapy.

Dr Hammerstein This demonstrates how difficult it is to precisely answer questions on this matter. Let us now turn to some vague suggestions of the past which never have been proved but still are alive in the thinking of some physicians. The older ones among you will remember that in 1963 there was a report suggesting, that if you administer oral contraceptives, fertility is increased thereafter.

Dr Diczfalusy There is an historical reason for this theory, which goes back to the original published paper by Rock, J., Garcia, C. R. and Pincus, G. (1957). *Recent Prog. Horm. Res.*, **13**, 323–46. As you know Rock was a Catholic and the only way Pincus could persuade him to participate in the study was by Pincus telling him that oral contraceptives would improve fertility through a 'rebound' phenomenon.

Dr Hammerstein In 1967 there was a theory put forward in this country that with oral contraceptives estrogen deprivation would develop, and even in the absence of any evidence this theory was reanimated 3 years ago.

Dr Hammerstein Furthermore, there was in the 1970s in our country an endocrine typology proposed. It was suggested that there is a progestogenic type, an estrogenic type, and an intermediate or endocrine-balanced type. Give the first one an estrogen type, the second one a progestogen type and the third one a balanced type oral contraceptive and all three will be happy. There is again no basic evidence whatsoever to support this well-sounding hypothesis. We should finally forget all of it.

Dr Breckwoldt I think it is very difficult, especially with the low-dosage preparations, to characterize the preparation as either 'estrogen dominated' or 'progestogen dominated' and for practical purposes such classification has no relevance at all.

Dr Hammerstein Furthermore, not long ago, we all more or less believed that postcontraceptive amenorrhea was a consequence of oral contraceptive intake. The incidence of this type of amenorrhea was not high, but it is only a few years ago that Nillius and Jacobs as well as others showed that there is no causal relationship between the incidence of postcontraceptive amenorrhea and the intake of oral contraceptives. Again we have learned that a long-established point has not stood the test of time.

A final point which I would like to mention here is the bioavailability of the contraceptive steroids. A recent study of Dr Goldzieher revealed that the pharmacokinetics of estrogens is different in different places of the world, and even within the United States. What are the factors which are influencing the bioavailability of contraceptive steroids? In the future this whole area needs more clarification, especially with regard to the developing countries.

Dr Irsigler I think you would like to make some comments about the use of oral contraceptives in young diabetic women.

Dr Irsigler This is a really critical issue and our attitude has recently changed concerning insulin-dependent diabetics. Until last year, it was recommended worldwide that the pill not be given because of the high risk of retinopathy and because the consequent increase in blood lipids increased the risks of an already high risk of micro-angiopathic arterial disease. We had always favored intrauterine devices for insulin-dependent diabetics, but there has been an increasing awareness that these devices are not very safe for contraception in the diabetic population. Diabetics are much more prone to infection and therefore run the risks of irreversible sterilization produced by an intrauterine device. They are often young girls and the nulliparous are not the best population for intrauterine devices. We have therefore changed our strategy, and now with the new triphasic pill, with its reduced influence on lipids and levels having no deleterious effect on glucose tolerance as well, we recommend this type of pill also for young insulin dependent diabetics. Vascular complications do not usually occur in the first 10 years of the diabetic's life and therefore we recommend the triphasic pill without contraindications (only if there is proliferative retinopathy would it be contraindicated, but you won't find it in the first 10 years). After 10 years, with the increased frequency of retinopathy it becomes more critical and it is necessary to keep a careful check on the eyes. We also recommend a time limit of up to 25 years' use of the pill. Afterwards most have had their children already or should have. If they have completed their family then surgical sterilization is recommended.

Audience member I come from Copenhagen. We have got a diabetes center and we have made a study with certain pill-using diabetics and we have not found any deterioration of their glucose tolerance. This finding is with non-insulin dependent diabetics that we have been treating.

Dr Irsigler Not only the type of pill has changed but also the type of pill-user has changed. They are younger, their smoking and possibly their drinking habits have changed, and our attitude to the definition of risk has also changed.

Most of you will know that the WHO recommendations, which define diabetes by oral glucose tolerance, were until a few years ago 160 mg/100 ml in the first hour by glucose load, and a 120 mg/100 ml blood glucose level in the second hour. Now the recommendations have changed and as a member of their study group I can say it was a considerable effort to answer the question as to what is diabetes and what is an impaired glucose tolerance test? Two years ago we defined that 140 mg/100 ml in the second hour is the beginning of an impaired glucose tolerance, (this was 120 before). If there is a 140 mg/100 ml blood glucose level after 2 hours (after a glucose load of 75 g) then diabetes begins with a 200 mg/100 ml blood glucose after 2 hours . Last year a British study showed that there is some risk if the blood glucose level is more than 90 mg/100 ml after 2 hours, but only for myocardial infarction; so the risk begins if normal values are not achieved after 2 hours. It slowly progresses and the real diabetic is in the range where more than 200 mg/100 ml is maintained. So this is also a change and we do not always know what to define as a true 'risk'.

Dr Wiseman 15 years ago everyone was very concerned about whether or not oral contraceptives could trigger diabetes. We have seen a lot of data today on insulin levels, and on the effects on glucose tolerance curves, and yet there is not really a well-documented case worldwide of any woman, despite these possible metabolic changes which have occurred, having had oral contraceptives trigger or cause diabetes. It is now very interesting to hear that there is general agreement in this conference that even diabetic women can safely be given oral contraceptives. I would say that the ideas today on metabolic parameters for coagulation and for lipids are at the same stage as perhaps we were many years ago with diabetes. We know oral contraceptives can cause minimal changes in a number of biological factors. We do not know what these mean clinically, and I would suggest that the mortality data which I have shown and from other data, that they are probably meaningless clinically. We don't know for sure and we will have to let time tell, whether they do have any significance at all. I agree we should measure them but I am not sure that we can interpret what we are measuring.

Dr Hammerstein Tables 2 and 3 give a summary of the clinically relevant benefits and serious risks of oral contraception. Note please that all the beneficial effects have been detected recently, i.e. shorter

Table 2 Oral contraception: protective effects

	Reference	*First epidemiological proof*
Benign breast tumours	Vessey	1972
Rheumatic arthritis	RCGP	1974
Adnexitis/Pelveoperitonitis	,,	1974
Ovarian cysts	,,	1974
Iron deficiency anemia	,,	1974
Ovarian cancer	Casagrande *et al.*	1979

than 11 years after oral contraception introduction. With regard to ovarian cancer a study of Casagrande *et al.* on 150 cases was reported recently where ovarian cancer was found to develop less frequently in women whose cyclic ovarian function had been interrupted by pregnancies. In this context the interruption of normal ovarian activity is one of the factors that may reduce the risk of ovarian cancer. Is there anybody who would like to comment on beneficial effects of oral contraception?

Table 3 Oral contraception: risks

	Reference	*First epidemiological proof*
Essential hypertension	Woods	1967
Venous thromboembolism	Inman + Vessey	1968
Cerebral insult	Vessey + Doll	1969
Gall bladder disease	Boston – CDSP	1973
Hepatic adenoma and hyperplasia	Baum *et al.*	1973
Ischemic heart disease	Mann *et al.*	1975
Subarachnoidal hemorrhage	RCGP	1977

Dr Breckwoldt I would like to refer to a recent paper that appeared in the *Journal of the American Medical Association* indicating that cancer of the endometrium and its incidence, was lower in pill users than in non-users and this decreased rate of endometrial cancer has been correlated to progestational compounds. Progestogen-dominated oral contraceptives were associated with endometrial carcinoma to a still lesser degree than estrogen-dominated compounds. There are two or three more papers confirming these conclusions, but I think we should be careful in considering these results and just take them as coincidence and not as causality.

Dr Hammerstein In any event, there are not only risks but also benefits from oral contraception and we may well find in the future additional ones from large-scale epidemiological studies or retrospective studies.

In Table 3 the more serious risks of oral contraceptives are listed, and again the majority of them have been detected only during recent years. With regard to liver tumors, I would like to report on a meeting in Berlin just a month ago at which occasion representatives of two large prospective epidemiological studies from England and from California stated that they have found only one such liver tumour up till now. On the other hand, in our hospital we have seen at least eight such cases in recent years and among these the majority were on oral contraception. Thus, it seems to me that there are special places where these types of tumors are more often observed and others where they are extremely rare. Even if their frequency is between 1 and 4 per

100 000 woman-years, as now estimated, liver tumor is something we have to look for. If you do laparoscopies for example you never should omit to look at the liver in patients who have taken oral contraceptives for a long time or who are still on the pill.

Dr Diczfalusy There is an on-going WHO study which is a case-controlled study co-ordinated by Professor Thomas from Seattle looking into the possible association between different types of malignancy and oral or injectable contraceptives. This study is to be published early next year.

Dr Wiseman To change the subject somewhat, one questioner has asked me 'what is the source of your data on oral contraceptive usage in women over 35 years of age?' The data I showed this morning is in fact constructed from two sources, depending on the year that I gave. The first year that I reported, which was 1968, usage was derived from the figure given by the Royal College of General Practitioners' study in 1973, and this showed that about 17% of women of that age group were oral contraceptive users. Since we know the usage of oral contraceptives in the whole population, we can therefore calculate what the usage in absolute terms was in that age group. It is an extrapolation admittedly from the Royal College of General Practitioners' data and may therefore, contain quite a large error. The second source was the 1976 data for oral contraceptive usage and this is from a paper by Dunnel which was published in 1979 from the Office of Population Censuses and Surveys. This actually deals with all the mortality data as well, that I was showing you this morning so it is pretty bona fide, but they are different sources and are therefore difficult to construct. Why I say that it is not terribly important if the Royal College of General Practitioners' data is inaccurate, is that in fact, as I showed this morning, the mortality rate would have to be doubled. Now if the RCGP's study was wildly wrong even then there would not have been a decreased usage in the older age group. What I showed was an increased usage, and the whole point of that was of course that I was looking for a counter-acting variable to try to explain why the mortality rate should go down, if oral contraceptives did cause ischemic heart disease. That was one bias I was looking for and I cannot find it, so even if the RCGP data is quite wrong and in error, there is still an increased usage in that age group and therefore that cannot account for the decline in mortality data. Another questioner said 'you showed a declining mortality rate while the number of pill users went up. Can you say some more about this figure, especially in connection with statements from other investigators from your country such as Vessey *et al*? I am not quite sure what the questioner would like to know here. I would suggest that the epidemiological studies that have been carried out by Vessey *et al.* and by the RCGP are looking at mortality data from a very narrow section of the population, i.e. that section that they have singled out particularly for study. I would suggest that the data I showed you this morning looks at the whole population in the United Kingdom and looks for trends to see whether the mortality rate has gone up, has gone down, or is stable. I would add that if the conclusions from the epidemiological studies are correct, viz, oral contraceptives do cause circulatory disease and do cause ischemic heart disease, then we should have seen in the mortality data that I showed you an increasing rate in those allegedly most at risk. We did not see this. We have actually seen a declining rate. All I have said is that these two data, (the epidemiological studies on the one hand and the mortality data that I showed you on the other) are inconsistent and if there were really a cause-and-effect relationship between oral contraceptives and circulatory disease, these two sets of data should be pointing in the same direction but they are not. They are pointing in opposite directions and therefore are inconsistent within themselves. Some studies show no increase in relative risk, others show three- or four-fold. The Boston study that I showed you this morning by Jick shows a 14-fold increase in rate, so they are inconsistent in direction and in dimension. They are inconsistent within themselves and they are inconsistent when we look outside these studies at mortality data as a whole. Another questioner said 'your investigation was based on mortality rates that says nothing about morbidity rates. Ischemic heart disease could still occur as a consequence of pill use but mortality could be low because of better medical care of circulatory diseases. I agree with that statement, I think that is quite right. I said nothing about morbidity rates because I have no data on this. What I do say is that if the epidemiological studies which have purported to show an increased relative risk for mortality rates, data such as I showed for mortality rates, which runs counter to their conclusions, then why should we believe the more difficult diagnostic criteria for morbidity rates? It is much easier to come to a definite diagnosis in a person who has died and has an autopsy and to say, yes that was a myocardial infarction than to say it in a patient who is in hospital and who may not have had an infarction. Now I do not know the answer to that, and at the end of the day all these data I have shown you, and that I have reviewed on the epidemiological studies are open to different interpretations and different conclusions, and which one you arrive at, which side you like to take, is a matter of judgement. One further aspect is the relative rates quoted for morbidity, and I would suggest that if there is a declining mortality rate, then it is a natural assumption. If there has been better medical care of circulatory diseases so that with increased morbidity there has been a declining mortality, because more lives are saved, I would expect that to be reflected equally in male mortality.

Dr Hammerstein We should now consider the problem of lactation and oral contraception, with regard to the developing countries which issue Dr Diczfalusy would like to comment on.

Dr Diczfalusy There have been a number of WHO studies and you may be aware that the last study did indicate that there is a significant decrease in milk volume even with combined oral contraceptives containing only 30 μg of ethinyl estradiol. It may be perfectly all right to prescribe such drugs in industrialized countries but I have serious reservations against their use in a developing-country setting by women who are breast feeding.

Dr Hammerstein Among others, there are two points we should also consider – one is contraception for women below the age of 20 and the other is contraception for those above 30 or 35. This is a long story. It started with the premise that there should be no oral contraceptives for young girls below 18, and then there was a stepwise decrease in the age. Finally we arrived at the conclusion that there is no harm to a girl even if she starts oral contraception soon after menarche. This assumption is based on the experience accumulated with tall girls who had taken high doses of estrogens or progestogens before the menarche for months or even years in order to reduce growth. Usually within a few months after stopping this treatment the first spontaneous menstrual period shows up, and after this a normal menstrual cycle develops. We now have more than 20 case reports on such women who have given birth to children later on. It was indeed a very unexpected finding that the menstrual cycle will establish in perimenarchal girls as soon as treatment is terminated no matter what the dose and length of estrogen and progestogen treatment had been!

Another question is when we do have to stop oral contraception in older women. Should we stop at 40, at 45 or at 50? I would like to know how the panel feels in this respect.

Dr Haspels If the four risks I mentioned this morning namely diabetes mellitus, hypertension, obesity or heavy smoking are not relevant there is no objection to giving the pill up to the age of 52.

Dr Breckwoldt At 35 years of age I re-evaluate the indications for oral contraception. It is well known that the fertility rate is decreasing by this age and there are other alternatives that can be used – for instance the intrauterine device which works perfectly well in this age group, so I try to persuade my patients to use this alternative. However, if the patient insists on staying on the pill for reason of its beneficial side-effects, I let her continue, and at the age of 40 I re-evaluate the situation once again.

Dr Larsson-Cohn I think the postmenopausal treatment must in some way come into this picture. We do give estrogens to postmenopausal women and we have not seen any thrombosis, but I think this is partly dose-related and I do not quite agree with Professor Haspels. I would feel that usually in the range of 45–50 or even maybe earlier, there must be ways of giving less steroid to these women.

Dr Hammerstein Before ischemic heart disease, and its correlation with oral contraception came into the play, nobody was seriously discussing when to stop oral contraception. After we had received the bad news from England (Mann *et al.*, 1975), and secondary to this the relevant warnings from the FDA in the United States and from other authorities, I personally followed these recommendations being convinced that there was some truth in the data presented at that time. From recent RCGP mortality data we know how the risk of oral contraception increase with the age of the patient independent of being smoker or non-smoker. If one prescribes oral contraceptives to women between 35 and 44 one should explain to the patient that according to Dr Larsson-Cohn she will take an additional risk of the same order of magnitude as the risk in car driving. It is, of course, then the decision of the patient to insist on the pill or not, however, I would not prescribe oral contraception to smokers beyond the age of 35 and to any other woman beyond the age of 45.

Dr Irsigler As an internist I would like to recommend you 'type' your patients not only according to smoking habits but also according to blood lipids, hypertension and their glucose tolerance. This should be the way preventive medicine develops in all countries – a test once a year, or be it every two years, and then you have a better background to giving the pill or not. We have an alternative now of changing patients from higher dose pills to the lower dose pills, and this should be re-evaluated about this age.

Dr Hammerstein We now recommend therefore the low-dose oral contraceptives for women above 40, and if there is a risk we can hope that the risk will be somewhat less with the low dose oral contraceptives, than with the traditional dosaged oral contraceptives. The pill we choose should have no or only low non-endocrine metabolic effects. On the other hand the endocrine spectra of the contraceptive steroids are of minor importance except for the antiandrogenicity, which may be beneficial in androgenized women.

Finally I would like to ask Dr Diczfalusy to tell us something about the future of contraception. After having talked about the sixties and seventies, what about the eighties?

Dr Diczfalusy I committed a grave error some 5 years ago in giving a talk on the future of contraception, and since then I have been nominated as a 'futurologist'. I can only tell you of new uses for old steroids, and these are mostly reflecting the needs of developing countries. The picture of what is emerging is that different countries and different geographical areas need a variety of contraceptive methods and in this regard the World Health Organization's Special Programme of Research, Development and Research Training in Human Reproduction specifically caters for the diverse needs of developing countries. One development is represented by vaginal delivery systems; these rings, which are now in phase III trials, release as little as 20 μg of levonorgestrel in 24 hours. There are many advantages to them; they are well tolerated and they can be self-removed at any time. The problem is bleeding. Biodegradable implants, which release levonorgestrel for 4–6 months, are also under development. Levonorgestrel is also available in the form of silastic implants, which have to be removed after a number of years, but have a life of 5 years or longer. There are new monthly and 3-monthly injectable contraceptives under development and at the same time some 'old-timers' such as Depo-Provera are also being re-evaluated. Hence in some developing countries at least, the future of contraception may be in a shift from oral to parenteral contraception.

Dr Hammerstein Let me finish this meeting with a consideration from the audience written down on one of these sheets. It reads: My suggestion for the title of the next symposium is '*Should* (and not *has*) the attitude change' and in addition 'my recommendation is that women users should be invited to speak and not only male scientists'. With these suggestions I give back to the organisers whose efforts to make this conference a full success are thankfully acknowledged.

Concluding Summary

R. Rolland

Our symposium on 'Benefits and Risks of Hormonal Contraception' has nearly come to an end. Since the introduction of oral contraceptives in the late fifties and early sixties continuous efforts have been made to:

(1) Reduce the estrogen content per pill.
(2) Reduce the progestogen content per pill.
(3) Switch to more specific progestogens with less side-effects, and finally
(4) Introduce the triphasic low dosage formula which has been the main topic of our discussion today.

In his presentation Dr Diczfalusy has given us some ideas of the tremendous work and the extremely high costs which are made before a new drug can be registered.

During the same decades as this development took place, a complete new generation of women has reached sexual maturity. For this generation the fact that sexual life and procreation are separated events has become self-evident. They have never felt the liberation from the (heavy) burden of procreation as have their mothers and this has in many instances changed their attitude to that of resistance against the oral contraceptives. As discussed thoroughly by Dr Hauser and Dr Evans the exaggerated reports in the lay-press on possible negative effects of the oral contraceptives, have even enhanced this resistance against the pill.

All of us have experienced the fatiguing discussion with women who are seeking our advice and for whom we are convinced that oral contraceptives would be the absolute best solution but who refuse to follow our advice due to the fact that (I quote) 'They say that the pill is dangerous'.

We all must try to rely upon data as presented here today in such discussions and translate them into an understandable language for our clients to convince them that the pill is safe. We have learned and I think it is quite convincingly demonstrated here today that the low-dose triphasic formula has little (or no) influence on blood pressure, renin angiotensin system, coagulation factors, carbohydrate metabolism and most of all on lipoproteins or lipid metabolism. We have also heard the reports on the clinical experience with the triphasic formula. As expected it gives a good cycle-control with endometrial changes more like the normal menstrual cycle, it has few, often minor side-effects.

In conclusion, with the introduction of this new triphasic formula with the concomitant reduction in progestogens per cycle a further step has made in the process of developing the ideal contraceptive with an outstanding cycle control and without (any) side-effects.

I thank all speakers for their contributions, I also thank the Schering company for the excellent organization and most of all I thank you in the audience for your contributions to the symposium. I also wish you a safe return home. Thank you.

Index

GPSR Compliance

The European Union's (EU) General Product Safety Regulation (GPSR) is a set of rules that requires consumer products to be safe and our obligations to ensure this.

If you have any concerns about our products, you can contact us on ProductSafety@springernature.com

In case Publisher is established outside the EU, the EU authorized representative is:

Springer Nature Customer Service Center GmbH
Europaplatz 3
69115 Heidelberg, Germany

Batch number: 10584446

Printed by Printforce, the Netherlands